Stress and Women Physicians
Second Edition

Marjorie A. Bowman
Deborah I. Allen

Stress and Women Physicians
Second Edition

Springer-Verlag
New York Berlin Heidelberg
London Paris Tokyo Hong Kong

Marjorie A. Bowman
Department of Family and Community
    Medicine
Bowman Gray School of Medicine
Winston-Salem, NC 27012
USA

Deborah I. Allen
Department of Family Medicine
Indiana University School of Medicine
Indianapolis, IN 46223
USA

Library of Congress Cataloging-in-Publication Data
Bowman, Marjorie A.
    Stress and women physicians / Marjorie A. Bowman, Deborah I. Allen,
authors. — 2nd ed.
        p.   cm.
    Includes bibliographical references.
    Includes index.
    ISBN 0-387-97319-2 (alk. paper)
        1. Women physicians — Psychology.   2. Stress (Psychology)   3. Women
physicians — Mental health.   I. Allen, Deborah I.   II. Title.
        [DNLM: 1. Physicians, Women — psychology.   2. Stress,
Psychological.   W 21 B787s]
    R692.B69   1990
    610.69′52′082 — dc20
    DNLM/DLC
    for Library of Congress   90-9788
                                                                            CIP

With 2 illustrations

Printed on acid-free paper

Camera-ready copy provided by the authors.
Printed and bound by R.R. Donnelley & Sons, Harrisonburg, Virginia.
Printed in the United States of America.

9 8 7 6 5 4 3 2 1

ISBN 0-387-97319-2 Springer-Verlag New York Berlin Heidelberg
ISBN 3-540-97319-2 Springer-Verlag Berlin Heidelberg New York

Dedicated to our families, particularly our children, Bridget, Johnny and Ted, the most important chapters in our lives.

Overview

This is the second edition of a book concerning the well-being of today's female physicians. The woman who chooses medicine as a career has a challenge that is in many ways unique, yet similar to women breaking barriers in other professions.

Today's increasing number of career and working women is an outgrowth of the women's and anti-discrimination movements which, however, have not yet freed the majority of women from their previous socialization as wives and homemakers. Many men, and women, are as yet unprepared for the major changes in the roles of women which have occurred in the last two decades. And it is the men, whose wives and mothers have held traditional roles in our industrial society, who presently are the mainstream of medicine. Women physicians, clearly the minority, are considered unusual anomalies and thought to lack impact on the whole of medicine.

The numbers of women choosing medicine are increasing rapidly, faster than societal norms and ideas can keep up with them. These women do not necessarily see themselves as feminists, or even as beneficiaries of the women's movement. But discrimination has existed, and will continue to exist, at least on an individual basis. Hopefully, however, the institutional barriers and myths are being struck down with the increased numbers of women entering the medical profession.

Women physicians--and the stressors they face--will change as the number of women physician increases, as women go from being a very small minority of the physicians in the United States to a substantial minority, perhaps even to an equal number. With security in numbers and more role models, women will feel less isolated, less 'on a pedestal' for all to view. While this will provide a positive influence, it will not remove the continued need for decisions and priority setting concerning personal life versus career, an issue men also face, but for which they have fewer expectations for participation in home-life and child-rearing.

Medicine itself is also evolving in structure, function and knowledge, creating a new world for all physicians and additional sources of stress for women physicians. Adjusting to these changes will require flexibility and responsiveness as well as leaders to mold the changes in ways that benefit health care providers as well as their patients. Women physicians will need to be forceful, willing and strong to carry forward their beliefs and to maintain or strengthen their standing in the world of medicine.

As long as there are women physicians, there will be women's issues, just as there are men's issues. Particular needs will change with time, external events, and women themselves. This book is intended as a still picture of today's women physicians, plus a time-eternal helpmate and thought provoker on dealing with the stress of being a woman physician in the 1990s.

The second edition is a monument to the current intense interest in the issues of women physicians. The amount of research and commentary that has been written about women physicians in the last few years has been tremendous, expanding our understanding of the role of women in medicine. This edition encompasses more up-to-date information, a new chapter on women as healers, commentaries and personal statements by interested individuals and expanded discussion in every chapter.

We hope and believe that this book will be useful to all women physicians and to others interested in female physicians or their issues and will provide as much of a learning experience for its readers as it has for its authors.

Marjorie A. Bowman, M.D., M.P.A.

Deborah I. Allen, M.D.

Acknowledgement

We would like to thank our many contributors, including the individuals who took time and thought to write commentaries for the book, those who read and critiqued portions of the book for us, and the many individuals whose lives and activities have provided ideas for this book as well as personal inspiration.

Contents

1
Historical Context

Women have practiced medicine for many centuries. In ancient Egypt there were many women students and women professors in the medical schools and, about 1500 B.C., both Moses and his wife were students of medicine (Turner). There has also been a long history of discrimination, recorded at least as early as 1421, when a petition was presented to King Henry V to prevent women from practicing medicine (Heins). The first formal degree awarded to a woman is said to have been to Constanza Collenda in 1431 (Nadelson).

Prior to the nineteenth century, the most common type of health care giver was the female midwife: labor and delivery were considered too 'dirty and debasing' for men (Fidell). It was not until the nineteenth century that men began entering obstetrics/gynecology in large numbers, and discrimination against women as physicians became powerful, vocal and open. An 1848 textbook on obstetrics, for example, stated that a woman's head was too small for intellect, but just "big enough for love" (Shyrock). Thus, it said, women should not practice medicine. Medical schools would not admit women. Harvard Medical School was going to admit a woman (Dr. Harriet Hunt) in 1850, but did not do so after the male student body protested strongly (Walsh). In spite of this initial rejection, Dr. Hunt is credited with being the first woman to successfully practice medicine in the United States, beginning in 1835 (Walsh), and became known as the "mother of the American woman physician." (Abram)

In spite of the admission of the first woman to a 'regular' medical school, Dr. Elizabeth Blackwell to Geneva Medical College in 1847, which many thought to be an accident (Abram), there continued to be a lack of opportunity for women in medical schools. As a result, three medical schools specifically for women were opened by 1864: one in Boston, one in Philadelphia and one in Cincinnati (Walsh). The first black woman physician, Dr. Rebecca Lee, graduated in 1864 from the New England Female Medical College in Boston (Abram). Medical societies, however, continued to refuse admission to women and it was exceptionally difficult for women to receive an academic appointment outside of a women's medical school. In 1867, the Philadelphia County Medical Society declared,

"We are not without very grave objections to women taking on themselves the heavy duties and responsibilities of the practice of medicine . . . man, with his robust form and trained self-command, is often barely equal to the task" (Coste). A year later, in 1868, Howard University Medical School was chartered and supported by the government to train black physicians (Abram). In 1870, the percentage of women physicians in the United States was only 0.8% (Heins), very few of whom were black or minorities. The relatively young American Medical Association (founded in 1849) passed a resolution in 1872 that said, "While we admit the right of women to acquire medical education and to practice medicine and surgery in all their departments, we deem the public association of the sexes in our medical schools and at the mixed clinics of our hospitals as impractical, unnecessary, and derogatory to the instincts of true modesty in either sex" (Weissman).

This entire era, and the long struggles of women to be accepted as medical students, interns and physicians is very well researched and recorded in three books: Doctors Wanted: No Women Need Apply (Walsh), "Send Us a Lady Physician": Women Doctors in America 1835 - 1920 (Abram), and Sympathy & Science: Women Physicians in American Medicine (Morantz-Sanchez). In order to have medical student positions, internship slots and thriving practices, women had to develop their own medical schools and open their own hospitals. Much of the thrust against women physicians was economically based (Walsh, Abram): most of the patients in the nineteenth century were women, and if they all chose to go to physicians of their like sex, the men would have more financial difficulty than they already did from an oversupplied field. But the work of a few women to be accepted was constant and ardent.

Some success was experienced when combined fund raising efforts, and a particularly large sum of money from one woman, created a $500,000 endowment at Johns Hopkins University in return for the equal admission of men and women, beginning in 1893. In spite of this, only 16% of the students were women in 1893-4 and 7% in 1907-8. Also in 1893, women comprised 23.7% of admissions to medical schools in Boston, 15.4% of those in Los Angeles, and 11.9% in San Francisco. By 1900 women constituted 18.2% of all physicians in Boston, and 42% of the graduating class from Tufts University. In the United States at that time, 6.0% of all physicians were women, or about 7,000 in number. Thus, some measure of success had been attained, although the advances for black women were smaller (there were only 65 black women physicians in 1920 [Abram]).

Women in the late nineteenth century brought domestic values to medicine (Abram) and emphasized preventive medicine which had been neglected by men. Many women physicians hoped that women would help upgrade a profession that had little legal standing and little prestige (Abrams). Women physicians worked with women and children, and some of the women physicians particularly claimed to bring special qualities to the profession of medicine (Walsh, Morantz-Sanchez). However, highlighting the difference in their sex was also used against them (Lorber, p. 20): "According to the Victorian stereotype, women were distinguished from men by their inability to restrain their 'natural tendency to sympathy' as men could and as physicians must" (Morantz-Sanchez, p. 26).

However, the success women gained by the turn of the century in increasing their numbers in the profession of medicine was temporary. For a variety of reasons, a number of the medical colleges created for women either merged with male schools or closed. Many men still did not want women in medicine. The editor of the Boston Medical and Surgical Journal felt that women physicians were an economic threat in a time of oversupply of physicians (Morantz-Sanchez, p. 53). Dr. Van Dyk, the president of the Oregon State Medical Society in 1905, claimed: "Hard study killed sexual desire in women. It took away their beauty, brought on hysteria, neurasthenia, dyspepsia, astygmatism and dysmenorrhea" (Bullough). Also educated women could "not bear children with ease because study arrested the development of the pelvis. At the same time, it increased the size of the child's brain and, therefore, its head. This caused extensive suffering in childbirth".(Bullough) In 1910, Flexner wrote in his famous report: "Medical education is now, in the US and Canada, open to women upon practically the same terms as men. If all institutions do not receive women, so many do that no woman desiring an education in medicine is under any disability in finding a school to which she may gain admittance. Her choice is free and varied . . . Women have so apparent a function in certain medical specialties and seemingly so assured a place in general medicine, under some obvious limitations, that the struggle for wider educational opportunities for the sex was predestined to an early success in medicine" (Flexner). However, the number of admissions to the male schools, many of which had become coeducational, did not make up for the loss of the women's schools.

Meanwhile, women entered other health fields, such as nursing and graduate schools in the health professions, in increased numbers (Abram). In 1910, women comprised 56% of the welfare workers and 30% of "keepers of charitable institutions."(Abram) Flexner, showing his own particular bias, concluded: "Now that women are fully admitted to the medical profession, it is clear that they show a decreasing inclination to enter it" (Flexner). The percentage of women physicians in the United States dropped to 4.4% by 1940 and did not again reach over 6% until 1950, after the influx of women medical students during the war years

(Walsh). Even in the mid-1970s, discrimination against women on the part of some medical schools was overt in the listing of their medical school admission requirements (Walsh).

There was a continual slow rise in the numbers of women in medicine in the United States from the early 1900s until another major surge in numbers started during the 1970s. In 1970-71, the percentage of women in medical schools was 8.9%, by 1975-76 it was 23.7% (Dube) and in 1988-89 37.1% of incoming medical students (Association of American Medical Colleges figures). American Medical Association figures for 1981 were that women comprised 12.2% of physicians, a rise in numbers of over 50% in the immediate prior five-year period (AMA Insights), and 16.4% by the end of 1988 (AMA Data Source).

These low percentages of women in medicine in the United States are not necessarily typical of the rest of the world. In 1965, most other industrialized countries had higher percentages of women physicians; in Germany, 36% of medical graduates were women; England, Wales and Scotland, 26%; and the United States, 7% (Facts on Prospective and Practicing Women in Medicine). The Canadian national average for first year women medical students was 37% in 1980 (Gray). Concurrently, however, medicine in the United States has a higher prestige level and more economic advantages than is true in many countries (Cartwright), and this may be one reason that men have fought harder for positions in medical schools and been less interested in women having equal ranks.

Women have, in spite of their low numbers as physicians, been the majority of workers in the health care sector, though the minority in leadership positions. "The occupational, class and sex structure of the United States health labor force is similar to the competitive sector of the economy (i.e., it is predominantly female, poorly paid and poorly unionized) . . . Upper middle class men compose the great majority of medical professionals, whereas lower middle and working class women form the greatest proportion of all middle level, clerical and service workers". (Navarro) Over 85% of health care workers are women (Brown), but the majority of decision-makers are men. This is also true within physician group of health care workers, where there are some women, but the vast majority of decision makers, high administrators and professional association leadership is made up of men. Women will have to do more than increase their numbers to have an impact at the leadership level.

Thus, women represent a growing minority of the physicians in the United States. Many battles have been fought in order to achieve the current standing for women, but inequality persists.

References

Abram RJ. "Send us a lady physician": Women doctors in America 1835-1920. W.W. Norton & Company, New York, 1985.

AMA Data Source. Women in medicine. American Medical Association, Chicago, Illinois, 1989.

AMA Insights. JAMA 1983;249(13):1703-1704.

Brown CA. Women workers in the health service industry. Int J Health Serv 1975; 5(2):173-184.

Bullough V, Voght M. Women, menstruation and nineteenth century medicine. Bull Hist Med 1973;47:66-82.

Cartwright LK. Conscious factors entering into decisions of women to study medicine. J Soc Issues 1972;28(2):201-215.

Coste C. Women in medicine: A progress report. The New Physician 1980:15-17.

Dube WF. Women students in the U.S. medical schools: Past and present trends. J Med Educ 1973;48:186-189.

Facts on prospective and practicing women in medicine. From a conference, Meeting Medical Manpower Needs--The Fuller Utilization of the Woman Physician. Washington, DC, January 1968:12-13.

Fidell LA. Sex role stereotypes and the American physician. Psychology of Women Quarterly 1980;4(3):313-330.

Flexner A. Medical education in the United States and Canada: A report to the Carnegie Foundation for the Advancement of Teaching. The Carnegie Foundation, New York, 1910.

Gray C. How will the new wave of women graduates change the medical profession? Can Med Assoc Journal 1980;123:798-804.

Heins M. Women physicians: They've come a long way, but what of the future? Radcliffe Quarterly, June 1979:11-14.

Lorber J. Women physicians: Careers, status, and power. Tavistock Publication, New York, 1984.

Morantz-Sanchez RM. Sympathy & science: Women physicians in American medicine. Oxford University Press, New York, 1985.

Nadelson C. The woman physician: Past, present and future. In The Physician--a Professional Under Stress. Callan JP (ed). Norwalk, Conn., Appleton-Century-Crofts, 1983:261-276.

Navarro V. Women in health care. N Engl J Med 1975;202(8):398-402.

Shryock RH. Medicine in America: Historical essays. Baltimore, Maryland, John Hopkins University Press 1966:184.

Turner TB. Women in medicine--A historical perspective. J Am Med Wom Assoc 1981;36(2):33-37.

Walsh MR. Doctors wanted: No women need apply. Yale University Press, New Haven and London, 1977.

Weissman G. Guilty with an explanation: Reflections on the marathon. Hosp Pract February 1980:121-126.

2
Women in Medical School and Academia

"A medical school in the United States is an inhospitable world for a woman." (Bowers) This quote from a 1968 article raises the following types of questions. If medical school is so inhospitable, why have so many women chosen this option, particularly in recent years? What happens to the women who so venture forth? Is discrimination so overwhelming?

The number of women entering medical school rose dramatically in the 1970s to the first year entry percentage of 37% for 1987-8 (Bickel). Over one-third of medical students are now women. Since the acceptance rate for women has not varied much from that of men for most of this century (Dube; Johnson 1983), part of the reason for the lower numbers for women must be lower application rates. If women were accepted at the same rate as men, why were not more applying?

Women Enter Medical School Because of Altruism and the Challenge of the Profession.

Women and men enter medical school because they have received encouragement from others, and see the profession of medicine as an intellectual challenge as well as an opportunity for helping others (the altruistic motive) (Cartwright). Consistent with this, women over 30 who applied to medical school were found to desire intellectual stimulation, competency and achievement (Kaplan). However, prestige and economic reasons rate lower for women than men (Cartwright) and in general are not particularly important motivations for women (Kaplan).

Women Who Enter Medical School Are Generally Outgoing, Independent and Well Adjusted, and Have Comparable Academic Records to Men.

Both men and women medical school applicants are dominant, achievement oriented, and autonomous (Rossler) compared to college men and women, or, as described in another study (Fruen) higher in "achievement, perfectionism, endurance, order and understanding, and lower in aggression, exhibition, impulsivity, play and social recognition." Personality profiles (Blakeney) of entering women medical students have shown them to be independent, socially outgoing, sensitive, concerned about others, optimistic, well adjusted, active and possessing a positive self-image.

It is generally recognized that the women accepted into medical schools are at least as qualified academically as men (Rossler, Fruen, Heins, Lindley), and perhaps, more so (Harward). One possible exception to this is their generally slightly lower Medical College Admission Test science scores (Rossler, Herman, Weinberg, Lindley) although Herman (1981) found this not to be true for women with science majors or for women in a special admissions program who were chosen for their abilities.

One of the Reasons for the Lower Number of Women than Men in Medical School is Pre-selection.

As noted, women have had about the same acceptance rates as men over this century. However, the percentage of physicians who were women in Boston at the turn of the century was about 20% (Walsh), a far cry from the 4-5% in medical schools in this country until the 1970s. Women apparently were not applying at the same rates as men.

The process by which women are culled out begins early in life. Sex-role socialization begins at birth (Crovitz). Women, in general, have lower evaluations of their abilities (Crovitz, Fiorentine). Many women who could be classified as potential physicians on the basis of high school grades and abilities do not even go on to college (unpublished, Sandra K. Wilson, American Institutes for Research, Palo Alto, California). This is partially confirmed by the higher percentage of women admitted directly from high school to a special combined undergraduate/medical school program (adapted from Herman). There is an equal ratio of men and women who enter college premedical programs (Fioretine), but women with moderate and low levels of academic performance in college are significantly less likely than men with similar academic status to apply to medical school, while those with high levels of academic performance apply at similar rates (Fioretine). Women medical students indicate that their parents were less supportive of their decision to study medicine than is reported by men (Bickel). Thus, many possible future physicians are turned away early or did not persist with their career aspirations. A societal influence has placed certain values and expectations on the role and abilities of women, which women, in turn, have internalized.

Subtle discrimination by medical schools could also be a factor. In 1970, the Women's Equity Action League filed suit against all medical schools, charging that they were discriminating against women, leading to low numbers of women in medical school. It has been suggested that, although the acceptance rate for women has been the same as men, women were better prepared than men (Norris). This, along with self-selection on the part of women students before application (Fruen) should have resulted in a higher acceptance rate for women than for their male counterparts. Women may need to be more committed than men to get into medical school (Matthews). A male ex-president of Women's Medical College has been quoted as saying, "You select your students on the basis of those you think are most likely to finish . . . If an effort were successful to get more women, it would mean that more men could not get in. The medical school people look at the fact that women drop out at a greater rate than men, but is that discrimination?" (Medical World News) In other words, possible women candidates have heard about the inhospitality of medical schools and decided not to apply; a subtle feed back loop to the applicant pool existed. Of note, however, women were admitted in greater numbers during the years of WWII--they were accepted in greater numbers when there were fewer men available.

Another interesting piece of data that lends some support to this hypothesis is that the personality profiles of women students did not change between 1969-71 and 1972-79 (Blakeney), the period of time when the numbers of women in medical schools increased dramatically. The author of this study notes, "Changing societal attitudes toward women's roles and the increased numbers of women admitted to medical school have not resulted in more diversity of personality types among women students . . . rather they have opened the door to larger numbers of women with personalities similar to those of women entering a decade ago."

"A number of medical schools may have 'secret' quotas" (Bowers). Whether or not such subtle discrimination could be proven, certainly the number of women applicants and students has increased dramatically in the ensuing years.

Women in Medical School Perform Academically Similar to Men.

Women perform similarly to men in the academics of medical school (Heins, Harward). They apparently do not do quite as well in the basic science years, which is probably related to their lower Medical College Admission Test science subscores (Weinberg), or perhaps because of lack of college courses in the same areas (Burke). Greenfield and Brown (1985) found no difference in Part I of National Boards by sex in their school's four year program. However, in the school's six-year program, the women were less interested in science and did not perform as well on the Part I of the National Boards, even when controlling for their similar SAT scores and college grades.

Women perform at least as well in the clinical years (Heins, Herman, Weinberg, Holmes). One study (Preven) suggests that women have better interviewing skills and another (Plauche) that they do better in ob/gyn clerkships. On the other hand, women rate the quality of their medical education as lower (Bickel).

Noncognitive rather than cognitive factors appear to be more important predictors of medical school achievement for women than men students (Calkins, Spiegel, Willoughby, Oggins). Oggins (1988) hypothesized that women should do better if the situation demands person-related tasks (such as in clinical clerkships) because of women's higher 'communal' orientation, i.e., motivation by social values, including helping, affiliation with others, and social involvement. Her data supported this presumption and found that men's clerkship written evaluations were better predicted by prior academic achievement and women's by their communal orientation. This was in spite of the fact that the women did not have statistically significant higher ratings for person-oriented values with the exception of 'work with people.' Oggins (1988) did not find that women's clinical grades were more related to social skills than men's, a fear which many women have.

Overall, the differences between men and women in academic achievement are minimal. Thus, once women are in, they perform as well as men.

Women Have Dropped Out of Medical School More Frequently than Men, but the Difference Between Men and Women Has Decreased to Almost Zero. Women Probably Drop out of Residencies Slightly More Often.

Students leave medical schools for both academic and nonacademic reasons. The net attrition rate for women was 3.01% and for men was 2.94% for those entering medical school in 1978-79 (Johnson 1983). In fact, minority women entering in 1978-79 had a lower attrition rate than minority men (Johnson 1983). Weinberg (1973) has found that women dropped out for academic reasons slightly more frequently than men. The overall dropout rate has decreased over time. The dropout rate in the 1920s was about 25%, but 15% from 1930 to 1946 (Johnson 1966). From 1949 to 1958, women dropped out at a rate of 16% compared to men's 8% (Johnson 1966). For this same time period, the academic dropout rate was slightly higher for women (7% compared to 5%) (Johnson 1966). The academic dropout rate continued to be higher for women through the 1970s (Johnson 1975).

Less is known about attrition from residency programs by women residents. Bowman and Allen (1988) found that women family practice residents (from a national survey concerning residents entering years 1980-81 through 1982-83) were slightly more likely to leave than men (14.2% versus 11.9%, odds ratio 1.22, 95% confidence interval 1.03 to 1.41). Women were more likely to leave for childbearing or rearing or spouse relocation (15.7% of the women who left) but men also left for the same reasons (total 5.0%). One internal medicine program (Freeman) found that men and women had similar overall completion rates (92.2% of the men, 89.3% of the women), but that women were more likely to have unexpected schedule changes (23.2% of the women, 12.5% of the men) and not finish on time. Thus, it would seem that women may have a slightly higher attrition rate than men from residency programs.

Women Choose Academic Medicine as a Career Slightly More Frequently than Men, but Advance in the Academic Ranks more Slowly than Men.

Women choose academic medicine as a career slightly more frequently than men (Langwell, Jolly). In fact, in the three years prior to 1981, 24.5% of those hired by medical schools were women (Higgens). The proportion of faculty who were women was 19.4% in 1988 (AAMC), higher than the percentage of physicians, about 15.3% in 1986 (AMA Center for Health Policy Research). Of 1961 U.S. medical school graduates in 1961, 10% of the men and 14% of the women were full-time faculty members in 1987 (Bickel). This is consistent with their trend toward choosing institutional settings for practice more frequently than men (see Chapter 5, Practice Chacteristics). The trend also may reflect societal permission to be a teacher (Abram).

However, women have infrequently reached the higher levels of the academic ranks (Bickel). There have been five women deans of medical schools in this country this century, one from 1982 to 1983 at Jefferson Medical College, which interestingly did not admit women students until 1961. A second was at Women's Medical College (now the Medical College of Pennsylvania) in 1955 (Farrell). The third is Dean of a medical school in Puerto Rico; the fourth began her deanship at Loma Linda in 1986; and the fifth was appointed in 1988 to the deanship at Albany. There have been no women vice-presidents for health affairs in this century (Farrell).

Nationwide, in 1977-78, 4.5% of associate deans, 9.9% of assistant deans, 1.5% of department heads, and 2.9% of division heads were women (Farrell). By 1987-88 (AMA Data Source), 11% of associate deans and 22% of assistant deans were women, a substantial increase in 10 years. Only 3% of department chairs are women (Bickel). Women are concentrated in the lower academic ranks (Jolly, Witte), making up only 3.5% of full professors (Farrell) in 1977-78, and 6.7% in 1988 (Bickel). Wallis (1981) found it took almost twice as long for women to advance up the academic ranks as for men at the four medical schools from which the information could be obtained (several schools refused to participate in the study). These same four medical schools had greater percentages of women than the national average, suggesting that other medical schools with less tolerance for women and lower percentages of women students would have worse records of advancement of women academicians. Lorber (1984 p. 47) also found in her sample that women had far less advancement even when controlling for achievement motivation, medical school performance, faculty and peer recognition in medical school, internship location and family responsibilities. Using these variables, only 13% of the variance in academic advancement for women and 14% of the variance for men was explained (page 47). Thus, most of the determinants of advancement are not based on predictable, objective factors.

Advancement up the academic ladder tends to depend heavily on publication, therefore studies of publication rates could provide helpful insights. Less publication means slower advancement. Two studies looked at different journals and noted participation rates of female authors compared to national percentages of women physicians. Matlin (1973) found no difference between the percentage of female authors or females accorded high status acknowledgments in the *New England Journal of Medicine* than national percentages. However, women are proportionately overrepresented on medical school faculties, thus this study actually suggests lower publication rates for women. Rosenblatt (1982) found similar participation rates for the *Journal of the American Medical Association* to national averages of women physicians, but proportionately lower numbers of women authors in the *American Journal of Psychiatry* and the *Archives of General Psychiatry,* compared to the number of women in psychiatry. They also found that women psychiatrists were more likely to publish articles in interdisciplinary journals (generally less prestigious) than medically sponsored journals. There appear to be no studies that look at the rates of submission to medical journals compared to acceptance rates, which would be necessary to know whether women actually submit as many articles as men. One step further would be to investigate the quality of the submitted articles, but this is indeed difficult.

Women are less likely to author a paper during medical school than men (Bickel). Female internal medicine faculty members are less likely to have research training, to spend time doing research, to have research grants, to have assigned research space or to author publications (Bickel). In contrast, a limited study of 1977-1981 graduates of Jefferson Medical College (Hojat) found no difference in the rate of authorship or presentation of papers or research, but did find that men were more likely to have developed medical procedures, instruments, drugs or techniques, serve on professional committees and receive professional awards or honors. A study of internal medicine women physician faculty members (Levinson) found a median of 6 publications in peer-reviewed journals; about half had published five or fewer articles. While there was no male comparison group, this suggests limited rates of publication for these women who were mostly between the ages of 30 and 40.

Thus, it would seem that decreased publication rates or less prestigious publications may be a source of the lower advancement in the medical academic ranks. Certainly, other factors can be operative, such as women's lower productivity in terms of the numbers of hours worked (see Chapter 4, Productivity). Women may also be less achievement or money oriented, therefore, less interested in doing the work necessary for advancement. Or perhaps, they have done the work, but not been aggressive or competitive enough to push their chairman to back their promotion. Discrimination, particularly in sponsorship for important positions or career-enhancing needs (Lorber) could also be a factor. Women also seem less interested in professionally related socializing, which may inhibit the development of sponsorship (Lorber). Academic women physicians believe having children inhibits career advancement (Levinson).

An interesting study of scientists may add some insight to what happens for academic women physicians. Interviews of scientists (73 women and 47 men) in the fields of physical, life and social sciences and engineering (Cole) found no difference in rates of publication by whether or not the women had married or had children. The sample was divided into the rank-and-file and eminent women scientists. Married rank-and-file women scientists in the sample, however, had lower publications rates than single rank-and-file women. Women married to scientists published 40% more than those married to non-scientists. For the eminent group of women scientists in the sample, the rate of publication actually went up in the three-year period around the birth of the first child. Overall, the men scientists published more than the women scientists.

One known reason for the lower percentages of women in the highest academic ranks in medicine compared to the numbers of women in medical schools is the long lead time before high academic rank is achieved. When the current influx of women reaches the lower rungs of the ladder, it will still be many years before the impact could be felt in terms of numbers of full professors.

Overall, it is likely that the slower promotion rate of women is multifactorial in origin.

Summary

Overall, men and women have much more in common in terms of medical education than they do different. Though women have fewer economic motivations for entering medical school, men and women are equally qualified to get into school, and do equally well academically. However, women with lower college academic records are less likely to apply to medical school than are men and non-cognitive factors are more important predictors of the performance of women than of men.

Until the last couple of years the number of women applicants had been increasing dramatically: they are now dropping, a few years after the number of male applicants dropped. While the numbers of women in medical school and practice continue to increase, "no male medical student has had to give up his seat to a women," as aptly pointed out by Pitts (1978). Women have essentially just taken up an increased percentage of the medical student slots created by expansion of positions in medical schools. It is unclear what will happen when medical schools decrease the number of available positions, as is occurring.

Women as faculty members tend not to be in positions of power, and to be concentrated in lower academic ranks, although they choose an academic career more frequently than men. The reasons for this are multifactorial. Hopefully, these differences between men and women will decrease as the number of women entering medicine increases. However, even with much effort, convergence will be a long, slow process.

References

AAMC. Faculty roster system numbers book. Association of American Medical Colleges, Washington, DC, 1988.

Abram RJ, ed. "Send us a lady physician." Women doctors in America 1835 - 1920. W.W. Norton & Company, New York, 1985.

AMA Center for Health Policy Research. Physician supply and utilization by specialty: Trends and Projections. American Medical Association, Chicago, 1988.

Bickel J. Women in medical education: A status report. N Engl J Med 1988;319: 1579-1584.

Blakeney P, Schottstaedt MF, Sekula S. Personality characteristics of women entering medical school over a 10-year period. J Med Educ 1982;57:42-47.

Bowers JZ. Special problems of women medical students. J Med Educ 1968;43: 532-537.

Bowman MA, Allen DI, Fini R. Family practice resident attrition: Reasons and rates by sex. Fam Med 1988;20(4):257-261.

Burke HB. Female frosh fare fine. JAMA 1986;256(24):3348.

Calkins EV, Arnold LM, Willoughby TL. Gender differences in predictors of performance in medical training. J Med Educ 1987;62:682-685.

Cartwright LK. Conscious factors entering into decision of women to study medicine. J Soc Issues 1972;28(2):201-215.

Cole JR, Zuckerman H. Marriage, motherhood and research performance in science. Scientific American 1987;256(2):119-125.

Crovitz E. Women entering medical school: The challenge continues. J Am Med Wom Assoc 1980;35(12):291-298.

Dube WF. Women students in U.S. medical schools: Past and present trends. J Med Educ 1973;48:186-189.

Farrell K, Witte MH, Holguin M, Lopez S. Women physicians in medical academia -- A national statistical survey. JAMA 1979;252(26):2808-2812.

Fiorentine R. Men, women, and the premed persistence gap: A normative alternatives approach. Am J Soc 1987;92(5):1118-1139.

Freeman RM, Waickman LA. Influence of gender on completing an internal medicine residency. J Med Educ 1988;63:914-916.

Fruen MA, Rothman AI, Steiner JW. Comparison of characteristics of male and female medical school applicants. J Med Educ 1974;49:137-145.

Greenfield B, Brown DR. Women and science performance in a six-year medical program. J Am Med Wom Assoc 1985;40(4):116-118.

Heins M, Thomas J. Women medical students: A new appraisal. J Am Med Wom Assoc 1979;34(11):408-415.

Herman MW, Veloski JJ. Premedical training, personal characteristics and performance in medical school. Med Educ 1981;15:363-367.

Higgens E. Women faculty members at U.S. medical schools. J Med Educ 1981;56: 202-203.

Hojat M, Gonnella JS, Moses S, Veloski JJ. Comparisons of male and female physicians on their practice patterns, professional activities, and perception of professional problems. Proceedings of the Twenty-Sixth Annual Conference, Research in Medical Education, 1987. Association of American Medical Colleges, Washington, DC, 1987.

Holmes FF, Holmes GE, Hassanein R. Performance of male and female medical students in a medicine clerkship. JAMA 1978;239(21):2259-2262.

Johnson DG. U.S. medical students 1950-2000. Association of American Medical Colleges, Washington, DC, 1983.

Johnson DG, Hutchins EB. Doctor or dropout? A study of medical student attrition. J Med Educ 1966;41:1099-1120.

Johnson DG, Sedlacek WE. Retention by sex and race of 1968-1972 U.S. medical school entrants. J Med Educ 1975;50:925-955.

Jolly P. Women physicians on U.S. medical school faculties. J Med Educ 1981;56: 151-153.

Kaplan LH, Pao M. Problems facing women students in schools of medicine, law and business. JCAH 1977;26:76-78.

Langwell KM. Career paths of first-year resident physicians: A seven-year study. J Med Educ 1980;55:897-904.

Levinson W, Tolle SW, Lewis C. Women in academic medicine: Combining career and family. N Engl J Med 1989;321(22):1511-1517.

Lindley D, Tudor C. Trends in medical school applicants and matriculants: 1978-1987. Association of American Medical Colleges, Washington, DC, 1988.

Lorber J. Women physicians: Careers, status, and power. Tavistock Publications, New York, 1984.

Matlin MW. Sex ratios in authorship and acknowledgments for medical journal articles. J Am Med Wom Assoc 1973;29(4):173-174.

Matthews MR. The training and practice of women physicians: A case study. J Med Educ 1970;45:1016-1024.

Medical World News. Women MDs joint the fight. October 23, 1970:22-28.

Norris FS. Statement before the Special Subcommittee on Education concerning Sec. 805, H.R. 16098, Discrimination against women in medical schools, June 30, 1970.

Oggins J, Inglehart M, Brown DR, Moore W. Gender differences in the prediction of medical students' clinical performance. J Am Med Wom Assoc 1988;43(6): 171-175.

Pitts FN. Women medical students. Letter to the Editor. JAMA 1978;240(12): 1238-1239.

Plauche WC, Miller JM, Jr. Performances of female medical students in an obstetrics and gynecology clerkship. J Med Educ 1986;61:323-325.

Rosenblatt A, Kirk SA, Koz G. The contribution of women authors to psychiatric and other medical journals, 1951-1975. Am J Psychiatry 1982;130(3):334-337.

Rossler R, Collins F, Mefferd RB. Sex similarities in successful medical school applicants. J Am Med Wom Assoc 1975;30(6):254-265.

Wallis LA, Gilder H, Thaler H. Advancement of men and women in medical academia. JAMA 1981;246(20):2350-2353.

Walsh MR. Doctors wanted--No women need apply. Yale University Press, New Haven, 1977.

Weinberg E, Rooney JF. The academic performance of women students in medical school. J Med Educ 1973;48:240-247.

Willoughby L, Calkins V, Arnold L. Different predictors of examination performance for male and female medical students. J Am Med Wom Assoc 1979;34(8): 316-320.

Witte MH, Arem AF, Hoguin M. Women physicians in United States medical schools: A preliminary report. J Am Med Wom Assoc 1976;31(5):211-213.

3
Specialty Choices
of Women Physicians

Why certain physicians choose particular specialties and others choose different specialties is somewhat of a mystery.   "Even the most sophisticated work has failed to account for the specialty of a majority of the sample".(GMENAC Staff Paper) When senior medical students were asked why they chose the specialty of their upcoming first year of residency, both men and women gave similar reasons (Cuca).   Opportunities for self-fulfillment topped the list, positive clinical experiences was next followed by the intellectual challenge of the subject matter of the specialty and the type of patient.   The two factors with the greatest difference between men and women were financial advantage, which was slightly more important to men, and type of patient, which was slightly more important to women.   Thus, men and women give similar reasons for choosing specialties, yet they choose different ones.

Women Choose Different Specialties than Men, Perhaps Because of Subtle Influences and Personality Traits.

The perceived 'femininity' of a specialty has also been suggested as a reason that women may choose one specialty over another. Certainly, the fact that women are in pediatrics much more so than suggested by their proportion among physicians would go along with this. So would the fact that they infrequently choose to go into orthopedic surgery or urology. One group of investigators (Beil) followed up on this by testing 68 men and women senior medical students with the Bem Sex-Role Inventory, a well-known psychological inventory of male and female traits on which one can score high or low on both male and female characteristics. The results were compared to the specialty choice of the student. Only in pediatrics and surgery were the results consistent with the hypothesis. 75% of the women who chose pediatrics scored high on femininity and low on masculinity; the other 25% scored high on both scales. Also, 40% of the men who chose pediatrics scored high on femininity and low on masculinity, 40% scored high on both, and 20% scored low on both. No women chose surgery, but of the men choosing surgery, 60% were high on masculinity and low on femininity and 40% were high on both masculinity and femininity. Of course, many physicians change their specialty choice after their senior year of medical school, and the results for practicing physicians could be quite different.

Another study provided an insight into one possible explanation for the different specialty choices of women. Ducker (1978) sampled 84 male physicians on the faculty of a medical school, asking them which specialties they would recommend to men and women, and why. The results, however unsurprising, are telling. The physicians, regardless of their own specialty, made recommendations differently for women than for men. Those specialties which they recommended were those which they believed offered opportunities for limited time commitments and which were believed to call for qualities attributed to women. For example, concerning pediatrics, the male physicians felt women were well accepted in pediatrics, could relate well to the patients and be sensitive to their problems, and the specialty required short training and was believed to be noncompetitive. In other words, women should go into pediatrics because they are noncompetitive and like children. "The fields most highly recommended were child psychiatry, pediatrics, psychiatry, and anesthesiology. The fields with the lowest rating recommended specialties were urology, orthopedics, neurosurgery, and general surgery."(Ducker) Faculty member perceptions of both the specialty itself and female medical students may influence specialty choice. Although faculty are not thought to be a major factor on students' specialty choice (GMENAC Volume 1), it is quite likely a subtle influence that permeates the medical school environment.

Women may also consider how the specialties are perceived. For example, socially, a woman urologist is viewed quite differently than a woman pediatrician. Our guess is that a women cardiovascular or orthopedic surgeon is threatening to potential suitors. Generally, women are expected to marry "up," someone with a higher prestige job and more income. There are not many careers or men who have a higher prestige job or earn more money than the subspecialties of surgery. Women who wish to find a mate may believe that their specialty will influence their chances of doing so. These fears have been at least suggested by Lloyd (1983) in her paper on how women medical students fear the impact of their choice of medicine on "their ability to find a romantic/sexual partner."

Personality is also a factor. McGrath and Zimet (1977) used an Adjective Check List to compare personality characteristics of women medical students at two medical schools to chosen specialties. They found the "future pediatricians and family practitioners were significantly higher than internists, psychiatrists and surgeons on personal adjustment, nurturance and affiliation." The group as a whole scored high on the need for achievement, counseling readiness, autonomy and dominance. However, the group's career choices were unusual (family practice was chosen by 44%), calling into question the validity of the study. This high percentage of hopeful family physicians may reflect the fact that the study was done on all four years of medical students, rather than in the last one or two years when more students have clarified their specialty goals. Calkins (1987) found that men and women who chose one of two specific specialties (family practice or internal medicine) were psychosocially similar, although the internist group differed in other respects from the family practice group.

Burnley and Burkett (1986), using data from a survey of third-year medical students, concluded that women who wished to enter surgery as compared to other fields were more likely to: 1) never have married; 2) have a physician father and homemaker mother; 3) have higher family incomes; 4) have chosen the profession of medicine earlier; 5) say that economic reward influenced their decision to enter medicine; and 6) agree that physicians need to sacrifice their personal lives for their work. They were less likely to believe that time demands of medicine were unreasonable. Both women and men students planning to enter surgery were more certain of their choice of fields, but the authors infer from the answers of the women that the women surgery students were even more career-oriented than male surgery students.

The higher percentage of women among foreign medical graduates also influences national statistics. In 1983, foreign medical graduates composed 21.5% of the physicians in the U.S.--19.8% of them were female; whereas, 10.5% of non-foreign medical graduates were female (AMA). Foreign medical graduates differ in specialty choices (Marder); alien foreign medical graduates were more likely to practice in pediatrics, psychiatry and pathology in 1986. One study suggested that foreign medical graduates occupied the lowest prestige positions, male U.S. graduates the highest, and female U.S. graduates mid-level positions (Goldblatt). With a higher percentage of women among foreign medical graduates, their choices, for whatever reasons, influence the statistics on the choices of women physicians. Unfortunately, there do not appear to be readily available statistics comparing the specialty choices of male and female foreign medical graduates to provide better data to test the strength of this hypothesis. It would appear, however, that the differences between U.S. and foreign medical graduates explains part, but not all, of the difference between the choices of men and women physicians.

Female specialty choices are negatively correlated with the potential income of the specialty (Marder). Rather than female physicians being "adverse to income, the findings most likely indicate that female physicians prefer specialties that have characteristics that are negatively correlated with income." Women are also less economically motivated.

Thus, in looking at the factors which influence specialty selection, the sex of the physician is the one that is most readily correlated with choice of fields. Women have traditionally chosen different specialties than men, particularly pediatrics and psychiatry. One study (Bureau of Health Resources Development) that reviewed the literature on specialty choice determined that the weight of evidence suggested that (1) personal economic factors seem to play a minor and temporary limit-setting role in specialty selection, (2) ability factors do not seem to be strongly related to the selection of particular specialties, (3) personality factors are major influences, but the literature on only three areas--surgery, psychiatry and academic medicine--was 'more unequivocal' than for other areas, (4) "Experiential factors, especially direct personal experience, are major factors influencing specialty choice," and, more importantly, (5) "While a variety of background variables have, in isolated instances, been linked to secondary career choice, sex is the only factor consistently correlated with specialty selection." The specialty choice is obviously multifactorial, but with major differences by sex.

Pediatrics, Internal Medicine, and General/Family Practice are the Top Three Specialties Chosen by Women, but They are Overrepresented in Certain Specialties and Underrepresented in Others.

In 1986, (see Table 3-1) the top seven specialties accounted for 66.8% of all U.S. women physicians: internal medicine 18.1%, pediatrics 15.1%, family/general practice 10.1%, psychiatry 8.0%, obstetrics/gynecology 7.1%, anesthesiology 4.6%, and pathology 5.9% (AMA 1987 Edition). However, this differed from male physicians only in certain areas. Women were overrepresented in pediatrics, anesthesiology, pathology, physical medicine and rehabilitation and psychiatry and underrepresented in surgery and family/general practice. In 1988, women comprised 16.4% of all physicians (AMA Data Source).

The Specialty Choices of Women Have Changed But Remain Different than the Choices of Men.

Not only have women physicians differed from men physicians in their specialty choices, they have also differed among themselves over time. Thus, in order to get a grasp on the specialty choices of women, one must

TABLE 3-1. Self-Declared Areas of Specialization for Selected Chosen Specialties for Men and Women Physicians in 1953, 1970 and 1986.

| | Percent Physicians | | | | | |
| | 1953 | | 1970 | | 1986 | |
	Men	Women	Men	Women	Men	Women
SPECIALTY:						
Anesthesiology	2.0	4.7	3.0	6.0	4.0	4.6
No Specialty	24.9	22.8	N.A.	N.A.	N.A.	N.A.
Family/General Practice	N.A.	N.A.	18.0	9.8	12.2	10.1
Internal Medicine	12.6	7.8	12.8	9.4	15.7	18.1
Obstetrics/Gynecology	8.7	13.0	5.7	5.3	5.2	7.1
Pathology	2.3	2.7	2.9	5.0	2.6	3.9
Pediatrics	5.2	17.5	4.6	14.8	5.1	15.3
Psychiatry	3.4	13.6	6.1	9.7	5.9	9.4
Public Health	1.7	4.6	0.8	2.2	0.3	0.5
General Surgery	17.1	0.9	9.5	1.2	7.3	2.3
Total	77.9	87.6	63.4	63.4	58.3	71.3

N.A. = Not applicable.

Adapted from Dykman RA, Stalnaker JM. "Survey of women physicians graduating from medical school in 1925 - 1940." J Med Educ 1957;32:3-38 and Eiler MA. Physician Characteristics and Distribution in the U.S. 1987 Edition. Survey & Data Resources, American Medical Association 1987. To make the figures comparable, Dykman's figures for gynecology, obstetrics and obstetrics and gynecology have been combined, and psychiatry and psychiatry/neurology have been combined.

look not only at the current specialty distribution of women physicians, but also look at the choices of the most recent graduates, see how the choices have varied over time, and how they differ from those of male physicians. How have the specialties of women physicians changed? In some regards, their choices are changing in similar ways to men physicians; they are also changing in comparison to men over the years. Essentially, as primary care specialties became more popular in the 1970s, they became more popular with both men and women, although women had always seemed to prefer primary care mostly because of their larger number in pediatrics. The trend toward increases in the primary care fields halted about 1976 (Steinwachs). By 1982, 41.8% women were in primary care (family/general practice, pediatrics or internal medicine), compared to 39.7% men (Eiler).

Langwell (1980) tracked all 1968 first-year resident physicians through the seven-year period from 1968 to 1975. She found that women were more likely to be in pediatrics, psychiatry, anesthesiology and a category called 'other specialties.'

The major change over time of the relationship between the choices of men and women is that there appears to be some convergence of the types of specialties chosen. This does not imply that there are no differences between current men and women. There are, but the differences have decreased. Based on national data of 74,625 physicians from seven graduation cohorts (1970 to 1976), Weisman and colleagues (1980) found a "trend toward convergence of male and female career patterns in several important areas: specialty choice during graduate medical education, patterns of switching specialties and subspecialization, and duration of graduate medical training." Also, "Male members of the 1970 cohort were most likely to conclude their graduate medical educations in internal medicine or the surgical subspecialties (excluding obstetrics/gynecology). Women were more likely to be in pediatrics or internal medicine. In the 1974 cohort, the most recent cohort for which data on the last year of training is available, these choices were still the most likely, although internal medicine replaced pediatrics as the most frequent choice among women."

As seen in Table 3-2, however, the choices of recent residents suggest there has been no major change in the last 10 years.

Conclusion

Women physicians, although frequently citing the same reasons for choosing their specialty as men, enter different specialties. The sex of the physician continues to be a strong determinant of specialty choice. Women have traditionally favored pediatrics most strongly, but also psychiatry, pathology, anesthesiology, physical medicine and rehabilitation and obstetrics/gynecology more than their male counterparts. These specialties do seem to be those which involve women and children or offer more regular hours in an institutionalized setting, which women have been shown to prefer. The specialties also tend to be ones for which long training periods are not required. They are also somewhat similar to the specialties chosen by foreign medical graduates, specialties which generally have lower prestige than the specialties chosen by men.

TABLE 3-2. 1978 and 1988 Specialty Choices of Women Residents

	1978 % of all women residents	1988 % of all women residents
SPECIALTY:		
Allergy and immunology	0.2	0.4
Anesthesiology	3.8	3.9
Colon and rectal surgery	*	*
Dermatology	1.2	1.6
Dermatopathology	*	*
Emergency medicine	N.A.	1.4
Family practice	7.9	9.8
Internal medicine	22.5	21.6
Neurological surgery	0.1	0.2
Neurology	1.5	1.6
Nuclear medicine	0.2	0.2
Obstetrics/gynecology	8.8	9.3
Ophthalmology	1.7	1.5
Orthopedic surgery	0.6	0.7
Otolaryngology	0.5	0.6
Pathology	7.0	3.4
Blood banking	0.1	0.1
Forensic pathology	*	*
Neuropathology	0.1	0.1
Hematology/pathology	N.A.	*
Pediatrics	18.6	14.0
Pediatric cardiology	0.3	0.2
Pediatric endocrinology	N.A.	0.2
Pediatric hemat/oncology	N.A.	0.3
Pediatric nephrology	N.A.	0.2
Neonatal/perinatal medic	N.A.	0.7
Physical medicine and rehab	1.4	1.1
Plastic surgery	0.2	0.2
Preventive medicine, general	0.3	0.3
Aerospace medicine	0.0	*
Occupational medicine	0.1	0.2
Public health	*	*
Psychiatry	10.8	9.0
Child psychiatry	1.7	1.6
Radiology, diagnostic	3.6	3.7
Radiology, nuclear	0.1	*
Radiology, therapeutic	1.0	0.5
Surgery	5.5	4.4
Pediatric surgery	*	*
Thoracic surgery	*	*
Urology	0.2	0.2
Transitional year	N.A.	1.5
* = < 0.01%		

Adapted from: JAMA 1980;243(9):877 and JAMA 1989;262(8):1033.

Differences continue to exist between men and women but appear to have decreased over the last couple of decades as the proportion of women in medicine has increased. The impact of changing choices on the overall specialties of practicing women physicians is not great.

References

AMA. Physician characteristics and distribution in the U.S. 1984 edition. American Medical Association, Chicago, IL, 1984.

AMA. Physician characteristics and distribution in the U.S. 1987 edition. American Medical Association, Chicago, IL, 1987.

AMA Data Source 1989. Women in medicine. American Medical Association, Chicago, IL, 1989.

Beil C, Sick DR, Miller WE. A comparison of specialty choices among senior medical students using Bem sex-role inventory scale. J Am Med Wom Assoc 1980;35(7):178-181.

Bureau of Health Resources Development. Medical specialty selection--a review and bibliography. U.S. Department of Health, Education, and Welfare, Public Health Service, Health Resources Administration, DHEW Publication No. (HRA) 75-8, 1974.

Burnley CS, Burkett GL. Specialization: Are women in surgery different? J Am Med Wom Assoc 1986;41(5):144-152.

Calkins EV, Willoughby L, Arnold LM. Gender and psychosocial factors associated with specialty choice. J Am Med Wom Assoc 1987;42(6):170-172.

Crowley AE. Graduate medical education in the United States. JAMA 1988;260(8):1098.

Cuca JM. The specialization and career preferences of women and men recently graduated from U.S. medical schools. J Am Med Wom Assoc 1979;34(11): 425-435.

Ducker DG. Believed suitability of medical specialties for women physicians. J Am Med Wom Assoc 1978;33(1):25, 29-32.

Dykman RA, Stalnaker JM. Survey of women physicians graduating from medical school 1925 - 40. J Med Educ 1957;32:3-38.

Eiler MA. Physician characteristics and distribution in the U.S. 1983 Edition. Survey & Data Resources, American Medical Association, Chicago, IL, 1984.

GMENAC Staff Paper Number 4. Social and psychological characteristics in medical specialty and geographic decisions. U.S. Department of Health, Education, and Welfare, Public Health Service, Health Resources Administration, Bureau of Health Manpower, Division of Medicine, Manpower Supply and Utilization Branch, DHEW Publication No. (HRA) 78-13, 1978.

GMENAC Volume 1. U.S. Department of Health and Human Services, Public Health Service, Health Resources Administration, Office of Graduate Medical Education, DHHS Publication No. (HRA) 81-651, 1980.

Goldblatt A, Goldblatt PB. The status of women physicians: A comparison of USMG women, USMG men, and FMGs. J Am Med Wom Assoc 1976;31(8): 325-328.

Haug JN, Martin BC. Foreign medical graduates in the United States, 1970. Department of Survey Research, Center for Health Services Research and Development, American Medical Association, Chicago, IL, 1971.

Langwell KM. Career paths of first-year resident physicians: A seven-year study. J Med Educ 1980;55:897-904.

Lloyd C. Sex differences in medical students requesting psychiatric intervention. J Nerv & Ment Dis 1983;171(9):535-545.

Marder WD, Kletke PR, Silberger AB, Willke RJ. Physician supply and utilization by specialty: Trends and projections. AMA Center for Health Policy Research, American Medical Association, Chicago, IL, 1988.

McGrath E, Zimet CN. Similarities and predictors of specialty interest among female medical students. J Am Med Wom Assoc 1977;32(10):361-373.

Office of International Health Manpower. Foreign medical graduates and physician manpower in the United States. U.S. Department of Health, Education, and Welfare, Public Health Service, Health Resources Administration, Bureau of Health Resources Development, Division of Manpower Intelligence, DHEW Publication No. (HRA) 74-30, 1974.

Steinwachs DM, Levine DM, Elzinga DJ, Salkever DS, Parker RD and Weisman CS. Changing patterns of graduate medical education. N Engl J Med 1982;306(1): 10-14.

Weisman CS, Levine DM, Steinwachs DM, Chase GA. male and female physician career patterns: Specialty choices and graduate training. J Med Educ 1980;55: 813-825.

Wunderman L. Female physicians in the 1970s: Their changing roles in medicine. In decade of the 1970s--The changing profile of medical practice 1980. Center for Health Services Research and Development, American Medical Association, Chicago, IL, 1980, p. 51-66.

"I'm tired of being first. No doubt there is a lot of glitter and notoriety that accompanies all this being the first female to attain a certain position, but after a while the pressure becomes enormous. The glitter fades and all that is left is the pressure. For once, I would like to be second or third. I find being first tiring."

Dr. Debbie Allen
Chairman of Department
30's, Mother of Two Pre-school Children

4
Productivity of Women Physicians

It is widely recognized that woman physicians work fewer hours than their male colleagues. Less clear, however, is the nature of the productivity differences between men and women, and how that difference is changing over time. Certainly, the fact that women physicians work less and see fewer patients is a source of consternation, and has led some men to believe that women should not be trained as physicians (Buchanan). Heins and colleagues (1978) quote a man as saying, "Women doctors do not practice enough to warrant training them,"--a major indictment. Two women, who are not physicians, estimated the dollar loss of the educational investment per female physician as $55,000 (Jussim).

Just what is the productivity of women in terms of hours worked and number of patients seen and how does it compare to that of men? The literature is somewhat conflicting on these points. Productivity can be reviewed in several ways. The most common is to look at the number of hours worked per week or per year. One can also look at the number of weeks worked per year, the number of interruptions in training or practice, full-time practice versus part-time practice, the number of months worked since graduation from medical school, or the percentage not active versus active in practice. All of these methods have been used, and all of the studies have weaknesses of one variety or another. For example, a study may only survey women without a control group of men, or fail to define important terms, such as 'full-time.' However, a review of all of the studies does provide us with some valid insight into the amount of time women work and how it has varied over the years.

The Data: Women Work Fewer Hours per Week and Take More Time Out of Practice, but the Differences Are Not as Great as Many Believe (See Table 4-1).

Studies of productivity have been based on nationwide surveys (AMA Periodic Survey, the Medical Economics Survey, Dykman and Powers), follow-up studies of alumnae (Johns Hopkins and Case Western Reserve, Harvard, Radcliffe College, University of California at San Francisco,

TABLE 4-1 Studies of Female Physician Productivity*

Productivity Measure: Study and Date	Percent Inactive	Percent Continuous Full-Time Since Graduation	Hours per Week	Hours per Year	Weeks per Year	Percent Full-time	Percent with Interruptions in Training	Percent with Interruptions in Career
Dykman 1953	12	49		1979**				
Powers 1964	10			1932				
Cohen 1973							'virtually none'	
Wunderman 1974	8							10
Weisman 1974							39	
Cartwright 1974								42
Mandelbaum 1975								
Heins 1976	16	59				76		
Hojat 1977-81	2		51.4			83	13	
Bobula 1978			44		46			
Mattera 1978			57					
Mitchell*** 1978-79			46.9		47.1			
Nadelson 1979	2							
Weisman 1980						79	9.4	
Lerner 1981			>40					
Silberger*** 1986			52.6		47.6			
AMA Data Source*** 1988			53.8					

*Further described in the text. The dates listed are for the actual survey or study, if available in the literature. Otherwise, the date of publication is given.

**Extrapolated from data provided.

***Only includes women physicians working at least 20 hours a week.

Jefferson Medical College), regional surveys (Connecticut, Detroit, and Philadelphia), and surveys of medical students (Jefferson Medical College, Georgia, and Michigan). All concluded that female physicians either work less or plan to work less than male physicians.

Nationwide Studies Larger studies probably provide more accurate data. The American Medical Association's Physician Masterfile is the largest single source of information on physician productivity. Wunderman in the Profile of Medical Practice 1980 (Wunderman 1980), using data from the AMA Physician Masterfile, reports that the percentage of female physicians who are inactive, defined as retired, semiretired, disabled, or temporarily not in practice and working less than 20 hours per week, has been decreasing. "In 1970, 12.3% of the 25,401 female physicians were inactive as compared with 8.0% of 45,540 in 1978." The greatest disparities in time worked were between men and women over the ages of 55. Of women ages 55-64, 12.3% were inactive, as compared to 3.9% of the men; the figures were 49.6% and 35.7%, respectively for physicians over the ages of 65. Over all ages, the figures were 8.0% for women and 5.9% for men; not a startling difference. Interestingly, the greatest disparities are not during the child-bearing years as might be surmised. This data is limited, however, because it does not provide more detailed information concerning reduced levels of work when someone is active more than 20 but less than 40 hours per week.

In a report from the AMA's Twelfth Periodic Survey of Physicians conducted in 1978 (Bobula), male physicians were found to work more hours per week (50.9 versus 43.7) and more weeks per year (47.1 versus 45.9). Using these figures, it would appear that women averaged 83.7% of the hours per year of men (2005.8 compared to 2397.4). In general, the differences had decreased from 9.6 hours per week in 1973 to 7.2 hours per week in 1978, almost entirely due to increasing numbers of hours per week put in by female physicians. During the same five-year period, the difference in weeks worked declined slightly, from 1.3 weeks to 1.2 weeks. The author believed that the productivity of women physicians was increasing and concluded, "Thus, it would appear to be inappropriate at this time to infer that the rapid increases in the supply of female physicians will have a signficant impact on either the organization of physicians' practices or the supply of physicians' services."

In another study using American Medical Association data, Weisman and colleagues (1980) found that among 74,265 physicians from seven graduation cohorts (1970 to 1976) the total number of months of gaps in training were almost identical for men and women for each of the years from 1970 to 1974, although there was a major decline for both sexes over that time period. The percentage of men and women who experienced gaps in 1974 was also very similar (9.4% of men and 10.1% of women).

Comparing data from the 1970 to 1980 Periodic Surveys of Physicians of the AMA, Freiman (1984) reported on the total hours of office-based physicians. Women physician's hours increased from 41.5 to 43.3 (not statistically significant) and men's decreased from 52.5 to 50.8, making the difference between men and women 17.3%.

More recent data from the 1986 AMA Socioeconomic Monitoring System (Silberger) indicates that women practiced 47.6 weeks per year, men 47.5. The women averaged 52.6 and the men 58.2 hours per week, with these differences generally consistent for all specialties. This suggests 2,503 hours per year for women and 2,765 hours per year for men, a 10% difference. The women averaged 99.3 visits per week (1.88 per hour), and the men 120.3 (2.06 per hour), a 21% difference. Of note, however, the SMS system only includes those who work at least 20 hours a week. By 1988 (AMA Data Profile), women physician hours had increased to 53.8 per week, men fairly stable at 58.7. The visits were 110 per week for women and 122 for men, a difference of 11%, indicating a decline in the difference between women and men.

Mattera, reporting on the Continuing Survey of the journal Medical Economics (Mattera), found that women physicians worked a total of 57 hours a week in 1978, while men worked an average of 62 (this includes all activities, patient care and administrative). This would suggest that women worked 91.9% as much as men on a weekly basis. The median number of patients per week was 84 for women and 124 for men, average 1.45 patients per hour of work for women and 2.00 for men. The difference in hours worked per week between men and women had held steady since the previous survey in 1974, but there was a slight trend for women physicians to devote more hours to professional activities.

These figures are similar to a Federal government report in terms of lack of change over time, but the visit-per-hour rate is different: the Third Report to the President & Congress on the Status of Health Professions Personnel (1982) reported that "there were only minor changes in hours worked by physicians and the average number of patient visits appeared to have declined slightly during the period." However, there did appear to be a decrease in productivity in that the visit-per-hour rate decreased from 2.58 in 1970 to 2.26 in 1980 for all physicians.

Mitchell reports 1978-79 data from surveys of the National Opinion Research Center for the Health Care Financing Administration (NORC-HCFA surveys). This study was limited to physicians practicing over 20 hours a week in office-based private practices with less than 9 physicians, thus generalization is limited. When adjusted for specialty, women averaged 46.9 and men 48.2 hours per week in patient care, a 2.1% difference. These differences persisted for all specialties, being most marked for psychiatry and obstetrics/gynecology; the exception was general practice, where women worked 53 hours to men's 49 hours. The women worked 47.1 weeks per year and the men 47.2.

Two studies of historic interest are those of Dykman (1957) and Powers (1969). Dykman surveyed every second women physician practicing in the United States who had graduated from U.S. medical schools between 1925 and 1940, and surveyed a like group of men. His study, however, is marred in several respects by the lack of comparability between the respondents and the nonrespondents. However, his studies suggested 12.4% of women were not working, and 68.0% of the women and 89.7% of the men worked at least three-quarters time in 1952. Almost one-half (49.1%) of the women had been in full-time practice only since graduation compared to 88.9% of the men. Dykman did not report the average number of hours of men and women, but determining group means for the frequency data he did report (and assuming that those 7.6% of women and 19.6% of the men who worked more than 3,500 hours per year averaged 3,750 hours), the women averaged 1,978.5 hour per year and the men 2,786.5, including those who reported none, suggestiong that women averaged 71.0% of the men. In 1964, Powers surveyed all women physicians who graduated in 1931, 1936, 1941, 1946, 1951, 1956 from U.S. medical schools, along with a corresponding group of men. Almost a tenth of the women were not professionally active. Women averaged 1932 hours of professional activity, men 2831, including those who were not active, suggesting women averaged 68.2% of the hours of men. Of particular interest, the percentage of women who worked only full-time since graduation increased fairly steadily from 36.6% of those graduating in 1931 to 49.6% of those graduating in 1956, for an average of 44.9%. Of course, this could mean that women tended to take breaks from full-time practice later rather than earlier in their careers, or that more of the women graduating later worked more. It is not conclusive that the percentage of women working full-time was increasing over the years, but suggestive.

Alumnae Surveys The following are the results of the alumnae surveys:

1. Lerner (1981) did a 34-year follow-up of women who studied medicine at either John Hopkins Medical School or Case Western Reserve in 1946. Of the 29 women for whom there were data, 23 (79%) worked full-time and 6 (21%) worked part-time; one woman had switched careers. The average workweek (including the part-timers in the calculation) was more than 40 hours a week.

"Only two of the 29 physicians had ever taken off more than 6 months. Time away from work following pregnancy was small and varied from none to 6 weeks."

2. Nadelson and colleagues (1979) found that of Harvard Medical School graduates from the years 1967-1971, 2.2% of the women and none of the men were inactive, whereas the graduates for the years 1972-1976, none of the women and 1.4% of the men were inactive. This study did not include hours worked, nor the numbers of patients seen. The cohort was young, and the levels of inactivity noted are similar to the younger age groups noted by Wunderman (1980).

3. Williams (1971) studied Radcliffe College alumnae who entered medicine from 1909 to 1967. She found that in the 212 respondents (84% response rate), "Approximately two-thirds of the group were working 35 or more hours per week; and a sizable number worked more than 60. Only a very small proportion (7%) devoted fewer than 20 hours per week." In a separate report (Williams 1978), it is noted that "the graduates from the 1930s and 1940s have practiced an average of 33 hours per week, those who graduated in the 1950s, 35 hours per week, and those who graduated in the 1960s, 44 hours per week."

4. University of California at San Francisco School of medicine graduates were the subjects of a study by Lillian Cartwright (1977). The 49 women respondents were divided into those who had received their training in a continuous fashion with no interruptions other than the usual vacations and those who had had interrupted (noncontinuous) training. Of the women studied, 30 (61.2%) had continuous training and 19 (38.8%) had noncontinuous training. Most interruptions (73.7%) were less than a year in duration. The continuous group was working 56.3 mean hours as compared to 40.6 for the noncontinuous group.

5. Hojat (1987) studied Jefferson Medical College graduates. The sample was 450 physicians (364 men and 86 women), who graduated between 1977 and 1981. 97% of the men and 83% of the women were employed full-time; 1% of the men and 2% of the women were unemployed. Males worked 59.08 hours per week and women 51.35 hours a week (a 15.1% difference).

Regional Studies Three studies in the literature report on productivity of female physicians in a region or area:

1.   Cohen and Korper (1976) surveyed 687 women physicians who
     were born since 1890 and who were or had been licensed to
     practice medicine in Connecticut; there were 373 respondents
     whose graduation dates spanned five decades. "Virtually all the
     respondents attended medical school and completed internships and
     residencies on a full-time basis."   More information on their
     productivity was not provided.
2.   Personal interview data obtained from 87 randomly selected women
     physicians and 95 men physicians in metropolitan Detroit by Heins
     and colleagues (1976 and 1977) found that 84% of the women were
     engaged in medical work at the time of the survey, 90% full-time.
     The graduation dates ranged from 1914 to 1971, with a median age
     of 46. "Only 7% were not working for reasons related to being a
     woman" (defined as related to children or marriage). Productivity
     was viewed in several ways: 90% of the working doctors were doing
     so full-time, 6% worked part-time but more than 20 hours a week,
     and 4% worked less than 20 hours per week. A 'Medical Work
     Ratio' (MWR), defined as full-time equated months in medical
     work since medical school gradution divided by total months since
     medical school graduation, was calculated. The mean MWR was
     0.88, and the median was 0.99. The mean for men was 0.993.
     "These statistics show that 83% of the women physicians worked
     75% or more of the potential time they could have worked since
     graduation from medical school." Only 9% of the women worked
     less than half of the potential time they could have worked. As far
     as career interruptions, 40% of the men had an interruption due
     to military service, and 13% of the women interrupted training for
     reasons related to marriage or children. Fifty-nine percent of the
     women had worked continuously since graduation. The conclusion
     was that "women physicians work nearly 90% as much as do men
     physicians." However, the MWR does not account for differences
     in the amount of work hours in a full-time week that other studies
     have found.
3.   Mandelbaum (1979) studied 71 women physicians selected from a
     population of 558 in the Philadelphia area in 1975. She found 40
     women (56.3%) she identified as Persisters (essentially those with
     cumulative nonwork histories equal to less than 1 year) and 31
     women (42.2%) identified as Nonpersisters (essentially those with
     cumulative nonwork histories equal to more than 1 year). Further
     measures of productivity were not utilized.

Surveys of Medical Students   At least three studies have asked medical students how much they expect to work after finishing their education:

1. Herman and Veloski (1980) analyzed data on career expectations of women who entered Jefferson Medical College in 1966-69 and 1970-73, for a total of 193 women respondents. "Among women who entered medical school in 1966-69, the mean estimated hours of work per week was 55, and that of men 59. Among students entering medical school in 1970-73, the average estimate made by women rose to 58 hours per week, and that by men to 63." Thus women expected to work less than men, but their expectations of hours of work increased from the earlier study group to the later study group.

2. Kutner and Brogan (1980) reported on the practice expectations of women and men students at the two medical schools in Georgia (Emory University School of Medicine, a private school, and the Medical College of Georgia, a state-supported school) in 1975-76. There were 262 subjects. The number of hours students expected to work were similar at the two schools, but the men expected a higher number of hours per week (range in means 58.0 and 64.6) than the women (range in means 51.3 to 61.5). Both men and women expected to work more hours than they would like to work. Women were more interested in the opportunity for part-time employment, and more frequently expected to interrupt careers than the men.

3. Rosen and collegues (1981) surveyed all four years of medical students at the three Michigan medical schools (University of Michigan, Michigan State University, and Wayne State University) in 1978. A total of 2,228 questionnaires were distributed; 962 questionnaires (43%) were returned. "On the average, respondents planned to work fewer hours (mean=53) than they thought, incorrectly, the average physician today works (mean=61) but slightly more than they thought the average physician should work (mean= 50)." The actual figure for 1975 was 51.8 hours per week. "Women planned to work significantly fewer hours (mean=50) than men (mean=53)."

The medical students estimated expected numbers of hours per week as higher than actually reported by physicians for similar years according to American Medical Association data. The expectations, however, were closer to those found in the Continuing Survey of Medical Economics, which are higher than those of the AMA.

Women Physicians' Work Hours Appear to Have Converged Somewhat with Those of Men, Partially Because Men Are Working Less, But the Differences Appear Relatively Stable in Recent Years. Women Still Average More Than a Typical 40-Hour Week. (See Table 4-2)

Many of the productivity studies are not directly comparable because of different methodologies. However, there is some evidence that women's work hours have increased in relationship to those of men. The two earlier studies by Dykman (1957) and Powers (1969) in 1953 and 1964 found female-to-male work ratios of about 71% and 68%, respectively, whereas more recent studies, such as Bobula (1980), Mattera (1980), Heins (1977), Silberger (1987) found 84%, 92%, 88%, and 90% respectively. Some of this would appear to be the fewer number of hours worked by men (2,786.5 hours per year in Dykman and 2,397.4 by Bobula), rather than more hours by women (1978.5 hours per year in Dykman and 2,005.8 in Bobula), although women may be working somewhat more (Bobula, Mattera, Powers). However, the work hours per year seem to be fairly variable between studies--men worked 2,764.5 hours per year in the study of Silberger, (1987) who only included women and men who worked at least 20 hours a week. Some of this is definitional, i.e., what is considered work, practice time, versus all time spent in related administration and educational activities. Thus, the productivity of women physicians in terms of average hours worked per year appears to be less than that of men, but increased in proportion to men since the 1950s.

TABLE 4-2 Women Physician Work Hours as a Percentage of Men Physician Work Hours*

Study and Year		Percentage
Dykman	1953	71
Heins	1976	88
Bobula	1978	84
Mattera	1978	92
Mitchell	1978-79**	98
Silberger	1986**	91

* See text for further description of studies. The dates listed are for the actual survey or study, if available. Otherwise, the date of publication is given.
** Excludes physicians working less than 20 hours per week.

Recent studies, however, while differing in methodology and in the amount of productivity, suggest that the differences have remained basically stable for the last several years.

Potential Reasons that Women Work Less Include Social Expectations, Stress, Children, Dual-Career Marriages and Personality Factors.

Since the studies generally indicate that women physicians average more than 40 hours per week, a traditional work-week in the United States, one can also question as to why the difference between men and women is even worth exploring. As long as they are working full-time or more, why should it matter?

Well, women do work less, although their productivity is increasing and the gap between men and women may be narrowing. There are some reasons and myths about this difference which gives us further insight into the women physician in the United States.

Children and household responsibilities immediately come to mind. "There is little doubt that fear of incompatibility of a medical career and a family turns women away from medicine." (Jussim) "Role conflict is the accepted explanation for woman's lesser participation in medicine."(Cohan). Decreased career aspirations and personality characteristics also may be factors. Stress may be a reason. One woman (Kinosian) wrote concerning her method for dealing with the multiple demands: "Guilt is nonsense and nonproductive. Obtain household help. It will be expensive, but a good assistant is worth every cent."

Stress Williams (1971) found that more than one-half of the married women physicians had undergone at least one critical period, and the most frequent response was to reduce career demands through decreasing the number of hours worked or by changing specialties. The next most frequent response was to withdraw temporarily from working. Both responses equate to decreased productivity. Stress apparently decreases productivity of women physicians.

Cartwright (1978) also identified three factors which accounted for the stress in a medical career for women, and therefore, could account for decreased productivity: 1) fragmentation: dual roles create greater responsibilities and conflicts; 2) internal conflict: 'femininity' and careers are often perceived to be at odds; and 3) nonsupportive external environment: a male-dominated field may not provide adequate support. Consistent with this, reasons that were cited by women for interrupting training in one study (Cartwright) were: husband's career and life course, child-birth and early child-rearing, homemaking, leisure, personal illness and disappointment with a training program (in that order). Of note, however, this study was of relatively young physicians, and did not include women in the older age groups which were identified as having the highest rates of inactivity in the AMA Physician Periodic Survey.

Children   How much a factor are children and associated home responsibilities? If children were a major factor, one would expect to see a greater concentration of decreased productivity and inactivity in the younger age groups. Williams (1978) had found that the younger female physicians worked more hours. This would be consistent with the findings of an increase in the hours worked by women physicians in the AMA Physician and the Medical Economics surveys, in that the recent influx of large numbers of women into medicine has skewed the working female physician population to the younger age groups, and the number of hours worked by women physicians overall is increasing. Heins and colleagues (1977) found that the months worked since graduation were inversely related to children, suggesting children were a factor in decreased productivity, but found that only 7% of the sample was not practicing medicine because of marriage or children. The age of marriage for women physicians is decreasing, and the age at which they have their children is decreasing (at least until 1973 when Cohen and Korper [1976] did their study of women licensed to practice medicine in Connecticut). Yet, young female physicians work more and have lower levels of inactivity than older women physicians. Almost 90% of male physicians' wives were either the sole or primary caretaker of their children (Nadelson), whereas it was rare for the female physicians' spouse to have the same responsibilities. (Weisman [1986] also found that 55% of married male physicians had wives who did not work outside the home; only 4% of the women said their husbands did not work.) Cartwright (1978) had found that those who went straight through training had fewer children. The study of Dykman (1957) in 1953 found that married women were more likely to have curtailed practice activity. This was reconfirmed by Powers (1969) among a 1964 survey, who also found that the greater the number of children the female physicians had, the lower the number of hours worked. A more recent study (Weisman 1986) found that single obstetrician/gynecologists worked more than those who were married without children (although this was not statistically significant) who, in turn, worked more than those married with children.

Mitchell's (1984) study using NORC-HCFA data found that children did not affect the hours or weeks worked by women. This study excluded those working less than 20 hours a week however, and may have excluded those who were mostly staying home to take care of children. In Working Woman's survey of 7,000 working women in the country, similar statistics were found: the salaries of women with three or more children were similar to those with fewer or no kids (Mann).

A study of women scientists (Cole) found no difference in the rates of scientific publications by whether or not the women had children.

Thus, children may be a factor, but probably not as much as many assume.

Dual-Career Marriages   Women married to another professional or someone who has a substantial income may not have as much incentive to make money and/or may continue to have sufficient household responsibilities to inhibit work outside the home.   Male and female physicians with outside income have been shown to work less (Sloan). The NORC-HCFA data (Mitchell) indicated that married women physicians (who worked at least 20 hours a week) worked substantially fewer hours per week (almost 3 hours) and fewer weeks per year, irrespective of the presence of children. The women physicians were less likely to increase work hours in response to income. This study also verified that women physicians with substantial non-practice income (such as from a spouse) worked fewer hours. Thus, being married and having non-practice income both were associated with lowered productivity.

Personality Characteristics   Various personality factors may be related to productivity.   Some people are just not interested in being workaholics, which many would call those putting in the number of hours male physicians do.   At least two authors have looked at personality charcteristics and how they related to continuity in training and/or practice. One of the authors (Cartwright) looks at continuity in relationship to hours worked per week briefly, whereas Mandelbaum only looks at continuity and not hours worked. Thus, their conclusions, however, similar, can maximally be generalized to the continuity in training and/or practice of female physicians and not to the productivity levels while working.

Mandelbaum's work is outlined in four articles (1976, 1978, 1979, 1979). She studied 71 women in the Philadelphia area through a combination of administered questionnaires, in-depth taped interviews, and Gough's Adjective Check List (ACL).   The women were divided into Persisters versus Nonpersisters (see above definition).   The Persisters were more likely to have considered becoming a physician prior to age 13 for superego oriented motives (satisfying parental desires and wishing to help others), were more self-confident, more self-controlled, better personally adjusted, more likely in the end to endure, to dominate and to achieve; they were more in control of, and accepting of self. "Those who persisted found medicine more salient than nonpersisters because of greater difficulties overcome in achieving the career goal; they preferred the role of physician to traditional female roles because of nontraditional feminine development" (Mandelbaum 1979 JAMWA:384-391). Nonpersisters were likely to have decided to go to medical school later for ego-oriented motives (independence and self-knowledge), were more individualistic and more inwardly troubled from multiple role demands, multiple goals and inner tensions. "When marital strains occurred, the Persisters were more likely to let the marriage go and to hold on to the career; the Nonpersisters more often accommodated themselves to the marriage (Mandelbaum 1978)."

Cartwright's work (1977, 1978) was based on studies of 49 young women physicians graduated from the University of California at San Francisco School of Medicine who had entered between 1964 and 1967. Her group was divided into two groups called Continuous and Noncontinuous on the basis of their educational training history. The Continuous group had no periods of time off from training other than normal vacations. Each subject was interviewed and took two psychological inventories, the California Psychological Inventory and the Adjective Check List (ACL). The Continuous worked more hours per week (56.3 compared to 40.6 for the Noncontinuous group), and were somewhat more satisfied with their careers. They had higher scores on two of six scales measuring interpersonal effectiveness, were more ascendant, forceful and confident. The Noncontinuous group were more like women in general on these items. The Continuous group were also more assertive and possessive of leadership qualities, but lower on the socialization scale, indcating less acceptance of conventional mores. The Continuous group was less 'feminine.' Similarly in the ACL, the Continuous group scored higher on self-confidence, achievement and dominance, consistent with Mandelbaum's findings for Persisters. Separately, Cartwright found that women who were high on both Career Satisfaction and Role Harmony were exceptionally confident, intellectually resourceful and tolerant. Overall, however, there was a high level of satisfaction for her study group (88% were either satisfied or very satisfied).

Thus, Mandelbaum's group of Persisters, who had less than a year's break since medical school graduation, and Cartwright's Continuous group, who had had no breaks in training, had similar findings on the ACL. They tended to be more self-confident, dominant, and highly achievement oriented. They were less 'feminine' by the usual definitions. These personality characteristics make sense as factors in productivity as well, and Cartwright had found that the Continuous group worked more hours. Productivity appears to be related to personality factors.

Other factors may be operative. Discrimination by patients and other physicians against women physicians and less interest in money by women physicians may be important determinants. These are discussed further in the Chapters on 'Practice Characteristics' and 'Women Are Different.'

Summary

Stress related to role demands, children, dual-career marriages and personality factors all appear to affect the productivity of women physicians. Women physicians, in spite of these influences, average more than a forty hour work week, but less than men in the same profession.

References

AMA Data Source 1989. Women in medicine. American Medical Association, Chicago, IL, 1989.

Bobula JD. Work patterns, practice characteristics, and incomes of male and female physicians. J Med Educ 1980;55:826-833.

Buchanan JR. The selection of medical students. J Am Med Wom Assoc 1969;24 (7):555-560.

Cartwright LK. Continuity and noncontinuity in the careers of a sample of young women physicians. J Am Med Wom Assoc 1977;32(9):316-321.

Cartwright LK. Career satisfaction and role harmony in a sample of young women physicians. J Voc Beh 1978;12:184-196.

Cohen ED, Korper SP. Women in medicine: A survey of professional activities, career interruptions, and conflict resolutions--Trends in medical education and specialization. First of two parts. Conn Med 1976;40(2):103-110.

Cole JR, Zuckerman H. Marriage, motherhood and research performance in science. Scientific American 1987;256(2):119-125.

Dykman RA, Stalnaker JM. Survey of women physicians graduating from medical school 1925-40. J Med Educ 1957;32:3-38.

Frieman MP, Marder WD. Changes in the hours worked by physicians, 1970-80. Am J Public Health 1984;74:1348-1352.

Heins M, Smock S, Jacobs J, Stein M. Productivity of women physicians. JAMA 1976;236(17):1961-1976.

Heins M, Smock S, Martindale L. Current status of women physicians. Int J Women's Studies 1978;1(3):297-305.

Heins M, Smock S, Martindate L, Jacobs J, Stein M. Comparison of the productivity of women and men physicians. JAMA 1977;237(23):2514-2517.

Herman MW, Veloski JJ. Career expectations of women and men in medical school. Letter to the editor. N Engl J Med 1980;302(18):1035-1036.

Hojat M, Gonnella JS, Moses S, Veloski JJ. Comparison of male and female physicians on their practice patterns, professional activities, and perception of professional problems. Proceedings of the Twenty-Sixth Annual Conference.

Research in Medical Education 1987. Association of American Medical Colleges, Washington, DC, 1987.

Jussim J, Muller C. Medical education for women: How good an investment? J Med Educ 1975;50:571-580.

Kinosian MJF. Letter to the Editor. J Am Med Wom Assoc 1979;35(12):462.

Kutner NG, Brogan DR. A comparison of the practice orientations of women and men students at two medical schools. J Am Med Wom Assoc 1980;35(3):80-86.

Lerner MR. The women: Who, where, when and why. J Am Med Wom Assoc 1981;36(1):5-12.

Mandelbaum DR. Toward an understanding of the career persistence of women physicians. J Am Med Wom Assoc 1976;31(8):184-186.

Mandelbaum DR. The nonpersistence of women MD's: A new diagnosis. Int J Women's Studies 1978;2(5):443-451.

Mandelbaum DR. Personality variables related to the career persistence of women physicians. J Am Med Wom Assoc 1979;34(6):255-259.

Mandelbaum DR. Education, medical training, and practice variables related to the career persistence of women physicians. J Am Med Wom Assoc 1979;34(10): 384-391.

Mann J, Hellwig B. The truth about the salary gap(s). Working Woman January 1988:61-62.

Mattera MD. Female doctors: Why they're on an economic treadmill. Med Econ February 18, 1980, 98-101.

Mitchell JB. Why do women physicians work fewer hours than men physicians? Inquiry 1984;21:361-368.

Nadelson CC, Notman MT, Lowenstein P. The practice patterns, life styles, and stresses of women and men entering medicine: A follow-up study of Harvard medical school graduates from 1967 to 1977. J Am Med Wom Assoc 1979;34 (11):400-406.

Powers L, Parmelle RD, Wiesenfelder H. Practice patterns of women and men physicians. J Med Educ 1969;44:481-491.

Rosen RH, Heins M, Martindale LJ. Practice plans of today's medical students. J Med Educ 1981;56:57-59.

Silberger AA, Marder WD, Willke RJ. Practice characteristics of male and female physicians. Health Affairs Winter 1987:104-109.

Sloan FA. Physician supply behavior in the short run. Industrial and Labor Relations Review 1975;28:549-569.

U.S. Department of Health and Human Services, Public Health Service, Health Resources Administration. Third Report to the President & Congress on the Status of Health Professions Personnel in the United States. DHHS Publication No. (HRA) 82-2, 1982.

Weisman CS, Levine DM, Steinwachs IDM, Chase GA. Male and female physician career patterns: Specialty choices and graduate training. J Med Educ 1980;55:813-825.

Weisman CS, Teitelbaum MA, Nathanson CA, Chase GA, King TM, Levine DM. Sex differences in the practice patterns of recently trained obstetrician-gynecologists. Obstet & Gynecol 1986;67:776-781.

Williams PA. Women in medicine: Some themes and variations. J Med Educ 1971;46:584-591.

Williams PB. Recent trends in the productivity of women and men physicians. J Med Educ 1978;53:420-422.

Wunderman L. Female physicians in the 1970's: Their changing roles in medicine. In The Decade of the 1970's--The Changing Profile of Medical Practice; Profile of Medical Practice 1980. Center for Health Services Research and Development, American Medical Association, Chicago IL, 1980, 51-66.

"When I decided in high school to become a physician, I never thought of it as something special; more as a way to fulfill my goals in life. Pursuit of these goals has sometimes meant that I have been treated as special or different.

From my own viewpoint, basically, I am a normal human being. Obviously not everyone sees it that way. One day a patient of mine said to my secretary, "But I saw Dr. Bowman in the grocery store in her jeans." Yes, I wear jeans. Yes, I go to the grocery stores. I, too, am human.

I like time with my family, to do everyday things. Read, play games, go to the zoo, roller skating, ice skating, Christmas caroling, playing family games, strolling the beach, attending church. I need all these things. I love life and enjoy all of it--career and personal. It means I'm busy, but I love it that way."

Dr. Marjorie Bowman, Family Physician
Chair, Department of Family & Community Medicine
30's, single parent

5
Practice Characteristics of Women Physicians

Now that we have seen that women physicians are different than men in terms of their productivity and specialty, it should not be surprising that their practices are different in location, type and resulting income.

Women Physicians are More Frequently in Salaried Positions in Institutional Settings.

Women physicians are less frequently in an office-based setting (AMA) and less frequently incorporated (Mattera).

Women comprised 15.2% of physicians and 27.4% of resident physicians in 1983 (AMA). Excluding residents, the following is the principal activity of physicians in 1986:

	% of Women Physicians	% of Men Physicians
Office-based practice	59.9%	69.3%
Full-time hospital staff	14.0%	9.0%
Administration	2.6%	3.1%
Medical teaching	2.2%	1.5%
Medical research	4.6%	3.6%
Inactive	10.2%	9.7%
Not classified/unknown/other	6.5%	3.9%
Total	100.0%	100.0%

Ogel (1986) found that men and women family physicians were equally likely to be in solo practice (25%).

The differences between men and women appear to have been in existence for at least 30 years. In 1953, Dykman and Stalnaker (1957) had found that 61.4% of women, but 85.2% of men were in private practice;

35.4% of women and 14.4% of men were in hospital, medical school or industrial salaried employment. In 1965, women reported to Powers and colleagues (1969) that 30.6% were receiving only a full-time salary, whereas half as many men (15.0%) reported a salary as their only form of income.

Expectations of medical students also seem similar to current practice patterns. Cuca (1979) found that more than half of senior medical students were interested in private practice, however, the interest by women was lower (54.3%) than that of men (67.4%); conversely, the women were much more inclined to salaried clinical practice (21.2% versus 8.7% for the men). Kutner and Brogan's (1980) survey of Georgia medical students found that women at the state school, but not the private school, were more likely to anticipate hospital-based practice or working in a publicly supported clinic. Women still seem to prefer salaried positions more frequently than men.

Another indicator of practice arrangements is the amount of practice expenses. Women physicians have lower practice expenses, with a mean of 33.3% of gross, whereas men had 38.2% of gross (Baum). The author attributes this to specialty differences--more women are in psychiatry and anesthesiology, for example, where practice expenses are traditionally low.

Women Physicians have Lower Incomes than Men Physicians.

In 1987, female physicians unadjusted net income for female physicians was 60.4% of males, $83,000 compared to $137,500 (AMA Data Source). The unadjusted net income per hour for females was 62-80% of males, depend-ing on years of experience, and the unadjusted net income per visit was 72-79% of males (AMA Data Source), depending on years of experience. More experienced women physicians had lower incomes compared to their male colleagues than less experienced women physicians. In considering specialty, the difference in the first five years in practice was greatest in surgery where women earned 47.6% of men, and the difference was least in pediatrics, where the figure was 94.6% in 1984 (Musacchio). In 1985, even after accounting for the number self-employed, the number of hours and visits, years experience, and specialty, women physicians still earned an estimated 12-13% less than men physicians (Silberger).

Looking back a few years, data from the AMA Twelfth Periodic Survey in 1978 (Bobula) found the mean income level to be $62,700 for men and $43,700 for women (69.7% of that of men). Taking into account the lower number of hours worked by women suggests they earned 83.2% as much as men, up from 75.5% in 1972 (using figures from Kehrer [1976]). However, the 1978 Continuing Survey of Medical Economics (Mattera) found the median incomes of women ($39,8230) to be 59.0% of the men's ($67,450). Klebanoff (1980) also quotes the Medical Economics Survey of 1973 as noting women's average income as $27,558, 57.5% of men's $47,945. This greater difference in income between the women and men in the Medical Economics Survey than in the AMA survey is particularly interesting since both the men and women surveyed reported a higher median number of hours worked per week in Klebanoff. Thus, amount of hours worked cannot be solely responsible for the difference between the two studies. Another, yet older, study from 1953 (Dykman) found large differences between women and men physicians--only 7.7% of the women, but 34.8% of the men were in the highest income bracket (>$20,000). Determining group means for the data would suggest that the women averaged about $9,720, 59.2% of the men's $16,414.

Thus, there does not appear to be any convergence between the incomes of men and women physicians (59% in 1953 and 70% or 59% in 1978, depending on the survey, 62% in 1985, 60% in 1987). Women earn less per hour and work fewer hours, thus have substantially lower incomes. Also, the difference between the incomes of men and women in medicine is not unlike, than the general full-time working public, where the ratio of women's to men's income varied between 59% and 64%, 1955-1970 (U.S. News & World Report), and was 64% for full-time workers in 1986 (Mann).

The Types of Patients that Women Physicians See are Different than Men Physicians--They Have more Women, Minority and Younger Patients in their Practices.

Consistently, women physicians have been shown to have a higher percentage of female patients than do men physicians. Kelly (1980) found that female patients were 1.49 times as likely as males to select a female physician in a Health Maintenance Organization; the women physicians' panels were 66.4% females, whereas the men physicians had 53.8% females. The women family practice residents in Bowman's study (1980) saw 73% female patients compared to men's 65%. The 1977 National Ambulatory Medical Care Survey (NAMCS 80-1710) found the average women physician's patient load to be 72% female while the average man's was 60%. Over the whole country, from the American Medical Association data, the figures are 62.4% female patients for women physicians and 59.5% for men (Bobula), not as great a difference as suggested by the other studies.

The race and age composition of female physicians' practices are also different. Bobula (1980) reported: "The percentage of patients who are white was 83.1% for male physicians and 77.5% for women"; and "The percentage of patients over the age of 65 was 30.5 and 25.0% for men and women physicians, respectively." In the NAMCS data (NAMCS 80-1710), minorities made up 19% of female physicians' practices, but only 9% of male physicians' practices. There was also a significant age difference in this survey: "36 percent of the visits made by patients over 50 years of age were to male physicians, compared with about 25 percent to female physicians." Further, "the median visit age of patients in the offices of female physicians in all specialties was 28.6 years, which is significantly younger than the median age of 36.8 years for visits to male physicians."

However, part of the difference in the race and age of patients is related to differences in specialty. When the NAMCS data (NAMCS 80-1710) was considered by specialty, the difference in race was most marked for general and family practitioners and internists considered together, but minimal for obstetrician/gynecologists and psychiatrists. The difference in age persisted only for general and family practitioners, but not for internists, obstetrician/gynecologists or psychiatrists. A difference in age was also found in a later 1980-81 NAMCS survey for general and family practitioners (NAMCS 83-1734).

Women Physicians have a Lower Board-Certification Rate than Men Physicians.

54.9% of all U.S. men physicians, but only 34.5% of women physicians, were board-certified in 1983 (AMA). 2.4% of men physicians and 0.8% of women physicians were dual board-certified (AMA). Less difference was found by Langwell (1980), where 39.6% of women and 48.1% of men physicians were board-certified 7 years after their first year of residency; this is probably because of the increasing trend towards board-certification in general. The 1953 study of Dykman (1957) had figures of 28.0% of women and 37.9% of men were board-certified, indicating consistency in the lower certification rate of women over the years.

Women Physicians Belong to Professional Associations Less Frequently Than Men.

Women seem to participate in professional socialization through organizations less frequently than men. Women seem to value this activity less (Lorber) and it often seems like a "third job" (besides family and work) for which they do not have time (Lorber).

These findings are consistent. In 1953, Dykman (1957) had found the women to belong to the American Medical Association (AMA) 82.6% of the time, the men 92.4%; women belonged to medical specialty societies 57.3% of the time, the men 64.5%. 30.5% of women and 45.7% of men physicians joined the AMA in 1988 (AMA Data Source).

In a survey of national medical specialty societies (Klos), only 14 organizations were able to identify their male/female membership. Twelve of the 14 had female membership of less than 5%. The two with a high membership were the American College of Preventive Medicine and the American Society of Therapeutic Radiology. Six of the 14 indicated that women had not held national office in their respective organizations during the last 10 years.

Allen (1989) surveyed all of the major specialty societies and found dismal rates of membership by women physicians. Only 20 of 41 societies could identify the gender of their members; only two of these (American Psychiatric Association and the American Academy of Family Physicians) was recruiting women and men at about the same rate. Of the 22 organizations that corresponded to a specialty board, 18 could identify their male/female membership. On average they recruited 60.7% of available physicians and 37.3% of available female physicians. The American Academy of Neurology only recruited 2% of the available women members. Nine of the 41 had special programs for women members; 8 indicated that no women had held national level offices in the previous 10 years; 3 provided modest financial incentives for dual career couples.

The identification of the women physicians seems even lower within a society geared specifically toward them--the American Medical Women's Association (AMWA). Only 8% of the women physicians belong to the AMWA (Morantz-Sanchez).

Discussion

Women physicians receive lower incomes and tend to prefer salaried, institutional settings more so than men physicians. Part, but not all, of the differences in income can be explained by practice settings, years of experience, number of visits, hours of practice, and specialty. These findings have been consistent over the last thirty years, although some of the differences between men and women may be decreasing.

Why would women physicians prefer salaried, institutional types of positions and have lower incomes? Obvious advantages of these salaried/ institutional jobs for women include relatively defined hours, greater job security and less long-term commitment. Better defined hours have clear advantages for child care. Women may also prefer the advantage of being able to quit at any time, such as when they have a child, rather than being tied to a private practice that may be difficult to leave.

Economic motivation is related to income (Erdmann) and is one factor in the difference between men and women physicians. Women physicians seem less interested in the monetary aspect of practice both in studies (Kutner) and anecdotally ("I never was able to bring myself to put a high enough value on my time and my experience.") (Dakin) Since the female physician is more frequently in a two-profession marriage, money may not be as much an incentive (Mitchell), and may actually be a disincentive in terms of taxes. Men may be more likely to charge more if they feel solely responsible for the income of an entire family.

Women may also choose lower paying academic medicine more frequently because of perceived societal permission to be a 'teacher.' Women are in the lower paying specialties more frequently than men. The three lowest paying specialties for several years have been pediatrics, psychiatry and family practice, the first two of which are more frequent choices of women physicians than men. Thus, women choose specialties which are traditionally lower paying, resulting in lower income.

Women may also value their home life more, or have more responsibilities at home (Mattera, Heins, Research Committee of the AMWA), and thus put less effort into their profession in terms of hours, board-certification, and professional associations. Consistent with this, in an AMA survey (Ad Hoc Committee), 92.7% of the women members described themselves as inactive in the organization due to other obligations, most frequently home and family responsibilities. Women may be less likely to belong to organizations if their physician husbands belong. Alternatively, Lorber (1984) argues that it may be thwarted career expectations that lead women to spend more time with their family and non-professional activities.

An additional possible factor for lower incomes which is not frequently discussed in the literature is discrimination against female physicians both by other physicians (Lorber) and patients. Referrals from other physicians are often necessary for both primary care and subspecialties, and women are less likely to be in the circle of referrals from other physicians (Lorber).

In terms of patients, Kasteler (1980), investigating attitudes toward women physicians in a Mormon community, found that there was no difference in attitudes among Mormons and non-Mormons and that half of the respondents had no preference for either male or female physician; but, of those who stated a preference, more preferred a male physician than a female physician. Attitudes of those who had seen a female physician were more favorable than of those who had not, and both younger and female patients were more likely to prefer female physicians. Needle (1977) also found that half of black college women had no preference for sex of their provider, and the remainder were evenly split on which sex was preferred. One fifth of a sample of female patients of both men and women physicians said they would not prefer a women gynecologist; 36% did not care (Haar). Another author (Adams), looking at the evidence concerning physician fees for procedures, found that the fees of women physicians were lower, and concluded that patients discriminated by paying female physicians less. An entirely different conclusion, i.e., that women physicians just do not charge as much as men physicians, which may well be the actual case, was not even entertained by the author. The author apparently overlooked the fact that the physician sets the fee, not the patient!

It appears there are some patients who definitely prefer male physicians and some that definitely prefer female physicians, but the number of patients who prefer male physicians is greater. As noted in Chapter 7 on Women are Different, the desire for a specific-sex physician probably relates to the type of patient problem. Experience seems to lessen this form of discrimination, so as the number of women physicians increases, more patients should have been seen by women, and become less biased against them. The fact that women are more likely than men to prefer female physicians is related to patient preference (or discrimination against males, if you prefer). A female patient may believe that a woman can be more empathic and understanding of her problems. Similarly, minorities, because of the shared minority status, may be interested in seeing a female physician. An alternative explanation for the greater number of minority patients is, however, that women more frequently work in institutional settings and publicly supported clinics, where minority patients often predominate, and women are more frequently in urban settings where they are a higher percentage of minorities.

Women probably prefer urban settings because of the social advantages. A single female physician may feel chances of meeting a suitable mate are greater in an urban setting. A married woman physician, on the other hand, is probably married to another professional, and has the constraints of a two-career marriage. In order for both married professionals to have satisfactory work settings, they must locate where more jobs exist, i.e., urban areas.

Summary

Thus, for a multitude of reasons, women are more frequently in salaried positions in institutional settings, have lower incomes, are more frequently located in urban areas, see more female, black and young patients, and have lower rates of board-certification and association membership.

References

Ad Hoc Committee Report on Women Physicians to the Board of Trustees of the American Medical Association, American Medical Association, Chicago, IL, 1984.

Allen DI. Women in medical specialty societies: An update. JAMA 1989;262(24); 3439-3443.

AMA. Physician characteristics and distribution in the US, 1987 Edition. American Medical Association, Chicago, IL, 1987.

AMA Data Source 1989. Women in medicine. American Medical Association, Chicago, IL, 1989.

Adams JW. Patient discrimination against women physicians. J Am Med Wom Assoc 1977;32(7)255-261.

Baum AZ. The wall crumbles ever so slowly. Med Econ February 18, 1980:104-107.

Bobula JD. Work patterns, practice characteristics, and income of male and female physicians. J Med Educ 1980;55:826-833.

Bowman MW, Gehlbach SH. Sex of physician as a determinant of psychosocial problem recognition. J Fam Prac 1980;10(4):655-659.

Cuca JM. The specialization and career preferences of women and men recently graduated from U.S. medical schools. J Am Med Wom Assoc 1979;34(11): 425-435.

Dakin TP. I chose a home-office. J Am Med Wom Assoc 1980;35(3):73-79.

D'Elia G, John I. Women physicians in a nonmetropolitan area. J Med Educ 1980; 55:580-588.

Dykman RA, Stalnaker J. Survey of women physicians graduating from medical school 1925 - 40. J Med Educ 1957;32:3-38.

Erdmann JB, Jones RF, Tonesk X. AAMC longitudinal study of medical school graduates of 1960. U.S. Department of Health, Education, and Welfare, Public Health Service, National Center for Health Services. DHEW Publication No. (PHS) 79-3235, 1979.

Haar E, Halitsky V, Stricker G. Factors related to the preference for a female gynecologist. Med Care 1975;13(9):782-790.

Heins M, Smock S, Martindale L, Jacobs J, Stein M. Comparison of the productivity of women and men physicians. JAMA 1977;347(23):2514-2519.

Kasteler JM, Humle S. Attitudes toward women physicians in a Mormon community. J Am Med Wom Assoc 1980;35(2):37-41.

Kehrer BH. Factors affecting the incomes of men and women physicians. J Hum Res 1976;11:526-545.

Kelley JM. Sex preference in patient selection of a family physician. J Fam Prac 1980;11(3):427-430.

Klebanoff S. Doctors do well, male doctors do better. Savvy February 1980:72-73.

Klos J. A survey of the national medical specialty societies. American Academy of Family Physicians Kansas City, Missouri, August 19, 1983.

Kutner NG, Brogan DR. A comparison of the practice orientations or women and men students at two medical schools. J Am Med Wom Assoc 1980;35(3):80-86.

Langwell KM. Career paths of first-year resident physicians: A seven-year study. J Med Educ 1980;55:897-904.

Lorber J. Women physicians, careers, status, and power. Tavistock Publications, New York, 1984.

Mann J, Hellwig B. The truth about salary gap(s). Working Woman January 1988: 61-62.

Mattera MD. Female doctors: Why they're on an economic treadmill. Med Econ February 18, 1980:98-101.

Mitchell JB. Why do women physicians work fewer hours than men physicians? Inquiry 1984;21:361-368.

Morantz-Sanchez RM. Sympathy & science: Women physicians in American medicine. Oxford University Press, New York, 1985, p. 342.

Musacchio RA, Willer J. Policy issues -- Income differences between young male and female physicians. Journal of Medical Practice Management 1986;1(4):223-224.

National Ambulatory Medical Care Survey, United States, 1977. Characteristics of visits to female and male physicians. U.S. Department of Health and Human Services, Public Health Service, Office of Health Research, Statistics, and Technology, National Center for Health Statistics. Publication No. (PHS) 80- 1710, Hyattsville, MD, June 1980.

National Ambulatory Medical Care Survey, United States, January 1980-December 1981. Patterns of ambulatory care in general and family practice. U.S. Department of Health and Human Services, Public Health Service, National Center for Health Statistics. Publication No. (PHS) 83-1734, Hyattsville, MD, September 1983.

Needle RH, Murray BA. The relationship between race and sex of health provider, the quality of care provided, and levels of satisfaction with gynecological care among black college women. Coll Health December 16 1977:127-131.

Powers L, Parmelle RD, Wiesenfelder H. Practice patterns of women and men physicians. J Med Educ 1969;44:481-491.

Research Committee of the American Medical Women's Association. Results of pilot survey of household help problems of women physicians in the U.S. J Am Med Wom Assoc 1972;27(6):324-327.

Silberger AB, Marder WD, Wilke RJ. Practice characteristics of male and female physicians. Health Affairs Winter 1987:104-109.

U.S. New & World Report. Closer: equality for women. April 3, 1972.

Wunderman L. Female physicians in the 1970s: Their changing roles in medicine. In Decade of the 1970s--The changing profile of medical practice; Profile of medical practice 1980. Center for Health Services Research and Development, American Medical Association, Chicago, IL, 1980:51-66.

As a child I was the target of more than one pedophile
  As a young adult I was raped
    I married an abusive drug abuser, a marriage now gone by

So I went into medicine
  I was bright enough
    I could help others -- prevent them from
      experiencing the pain I had felt

It has taken years
  but gradually my mental health has improved
    my goals have not shifted

Medicine offers wonderful opportunities to help others
    physically and emotionally
        I love it

                    anonymous practicing woman physician

6
Mental Health Status
of Women Physicians

Physicians lead lives that contain many potentially stressful components. Long work hours, open-ended time schedules, night calls with associated sleep deprivation, dealing with death and dying and other emotional aspects of people's lives--all can be stressful. On the other side of the coin, physicians tend to make more money than the average person have greater prestige and have the opportunity to help many people. The balance of these two sides of the equation varies according to the individual physician. For one physician, the stresses might seem dominant, for another, the benefits more important.

Generally, however, what are the overall effects? Are physicians *in toto* more stressed than the general public? Are women physicians more stressed than other working women? And, are female physicians even worse off than their medical male counterparts by having the additional stressors of family/career conflict or sexual discrimination? Several measures can be employed to assess the balance. Frequently considered are the incidence of mental illness, alcohol and drug abuse, suicide, and bad marriages. In this chapter, the evidence will be reviewed, and some generalizations will be attempted.

It must be remembered that the relationship between stress and the development of psychiatric illness is not fully clear. Andrews and Tennant (1978) argue that stressful life events may account for as little as 10% of psychiatric illness. Cooke and Hole (1983) believe it to be closer to one-third of psychiatric cases. Certainly genetics and other environmental factors must be involved in the development of psychiatric illness. Nevertheless, it is widely believed that stress can precipitate psychiatric illness, particularly depression.

Physicians Have Slightly Lower Death Rates than the Average
Citizen, Particularly from Accidents, but More Frequently
Commit Suicide. Female Physicians Commit Suicide More
Frequently than Females in the Population, but Probably at
About the Same Rate as Male Physicians Do.

Trying to review the literature on physician death and suicide rates is
frustrating. There are few recent studies, and mortality statistics vary
significantly over time. Additionally, the methodologies used are of only
fair quality. Threatening any attempts at generalization is the fact that
death certificates are an uncertain and probably uneven form of
determining death rates from specific causes (Annotated Bibliography,
Pollock, Kircher), yet the alternate study methodology of intimate
knowledge of a small local population tends to provide too few cases.
Physicians who fill out death certificates may 'hide' the suicides of their
fellow physicians under euphemistic terms, just as they tend not to list
'alcohol' as a contributing cause on the death certificates of U.S. Army
veterans who die of trauma (Pollock).

The American Medical Association attempts to list and determine the
causes of deaths for all physicians through news clippings, notification from
relatives, and sometimes by death certificates. The problems with this
methodology have been outlined (Rose 1973), and the error rate may be
high. Comparing this data base to general population data bases presents
another problem, since causes of the physician deaths are then much more
closely reviewed than those of the general population as determined solely
from death certificates.

The available physician suicide and mortality studies are outlined in
Table 6-1.

The earliest mention of physician suicides in this century appears to be
an editorial in *JAMA* (Anonymous) in 1903 which noted that the 519
physician 'self-murders' in the previous 12 1/2 years was excessive, and
blamed the excess on the overcrowding of the profession--there were just
too many physicians for the population size. Of the more recent studies,
one of the better methodologically is that of Rose and Rosow (1973), who
used death certificates in California to review the physician suicide rate.
California physicians were required to report all suicides, and the coroners
investigated each. Thus, hopefully, the suicide rate would be relatively
accurate. The suicide data was also age-adjusted, which is necessary in
suicide studies because suicides tend to increase in older age groups. Of
406,498 deaths from 1959 to 1961, the male physician suicide rate was
79/100,000, higher than the general population average of 38/100,000 and

TABLE 6-1 Physician Suicide and Mortality Studies

Author	Basic Population and Year	Method	Suicide Rate	# of Suicides	Suicide Preference	Comment	Methodologic Comments
Anonymous	U.S. deaths previous 12½ years prior to 1903	Unclear	519 physician suicides "higher than general public	519		High suicide rate attributed to competition among excess number of physicians	Not enough information to ascertain
Emerson H, et al	U.S. white male, physician deaths 1925	AMA data	Suicide 45.4/100,000; overall death rate less than expected	61		↑ heart disease ↑ pneumonia ↑ diabetes ↓ chronic nephritis and Bright's disease, violence, typhoid fever, TB, cancer	AMA data (see text)
Dublin L, et al	U.S. physician deaths 1938-42 suicides equal 1.04	AMA data	Suicide 39.0/100,000 actual/expected	?		↑ heart disease ↑ diabetes, cirrhosis ↓ accidents (0.89) ↓ other (0.60)	AMA data see text)
Williams SV, et al	199 deaths of 1193 graduates of Harvard Medical School 1923-24, 1932-34, 1942-44; males <1% nonwhite; all deaths by 1970	Alumni files; Cohort study	Consistently lower mortality from all causes than national data		Medical specialties > surgical specialties	Cohort study-manipulation necessary to make national data compatible. Specific causes of death not investigated	Small sample size

TABLE 6-1 (Continued)

Author	Basic Population and Year	Method	Suicide Rate	# of Suicides	Suicide Preference	Comment	Methodologic Comments
Thomas CB	1337 Hopkins Medical students classes 1948-64; data collection 1969	Death certificates and other direct information	14/1337 suicides =1.04% 17/1337 other deaths =1.27%	14			Small sample size
Bruce DL, et al	U.S. Anesthesiologist deaths male, 1947-66	AMA data plus	441 deaths; 7.9% suicides, suicide rate 2.20 X 1947-56 population, 2.86 X 1957-66 population. Overall death rate 1.22 X U.S. population 1947-56; 1.44 X 1957-1966	35		↓ lung cancer, coronary artery disease, accidents ↑ suicide and malignancies of lymphoid and reticulo endothelial tissues	AMA data (see text)
Dickinson FG, et al	U.S. 10,738 physician deaths assumed all male 1949-51	AMA files and death certificates (all except 175 confirmed by both); age-adjusted	Actual/expected deaths=0.93 Actual/expected suicides=1.03	1908		↑ heart disease ↑ diabetes ↑ suicide ↓ cirrhosis ↓ accidents	AMA data (see text)

TABLE 6-1 (Continued)

Author	Basic Population and Year	Method	Suicide Rate	# of Suicides	Suicide Preference	Comment	Methodologic Problems
Blachly PH, et al	Oregon suicides 1950-61	Death certificates White collar 15/100,000	♂ physicians 30/100,000	8 ♂ physicians			Low number of cases
Doll R, et al	British white male physicians 1951-71	British death certificates 0.7% poisoning; 2.38% trauma	1.72% deaths from suicide;	173	General practitioners	Total deaths related to cigarette smoking	
Rose KD, et al California	All deaths (406,498) 1959-61	Death certificates	♂ physicians 79/100,000 ♀ health care professionals 33/100,000			Physicians required by law to report suicides and all are investigated by coroner. Suicide in physicians related to age and divorce	Insufficient numbers of female physician suicides to ascertain rates
Blachly PH, et al	U.S. physician 5/65 - 11/67	JAMA obituary columns; surveyed survivors	2.66% of deaths 74/100,000 estimated from Figure 1	200	Psychiatry, ophthalmology, ENT, anesthesiology over represented	Many had mental health problems	AMA data inconsistent number suicides noted - 200 or 249?

TABLE 6-1 (Continued)

Author	Basic Population and Year	Method	Suicide Rate	# of Suicides	Suicide Preference	Comment	Methodologic Comments
DeSole DE, et al	U.S. physician deaths 5/65 - 5/68	JAMA obituaries with personal follow-up	33/100,000	291	Psychiatry, ENT, anesthesiology, ophthalmology	36% used drugs (general population 13%)	AMA data
Steppacher RC, et al	U.S. physician deaths 1965-70	AMA data plus confirmation; age adjusted	♂ 1.15 X population 30.9/100,000 ♀ 3 X population 33.6/100,000	489 ♂ physicians 41 ♀ physicians		20% ♀ suicides were during training ♂ suicide highest age 45-64. ♀ 75.6% drugs. ♂ physicians 38.2% drugs, 39.1% guns. "Conservative in suicide determination"	
Craig AG, et al	U.S. physician deaths 1965-67	AMA data plus follow-up	♂ physicians 28.3/100,000 (2.61%) ♀ physicians 40.5/100,000	211 ♂ physician suicides 17 ♀ physician suicides	High in otolaryngologists		AMA data see text). Low #'s of suicides. not age-adjusted
Pitts FN Jr, et al	U.S. female physician deaths 1967-72	AMA records	♀ physicians 40.7/100,000 ♀ population 11.4/100,000	49		71% ♀ physicians used drugs/ 8 were in training	Not age-adjusted AMA data

TABLE 6-1 (Continued)

Author	Basic Population and Year	Method	Suicide Rate	# of Suicides	Suicide Preference	Comment	Methodologic Comments
Rich CL, Pitts FN	U.S. physician deaths 1967-72	AMA records	♀ physicians 40.7/100,000 ♂ physicians 39.7/100,000 physician suicides	49 ♀ physician suicides 544 ♂	High in psychiatrists		Not age-AMA data
Goodman LJ	All U.S. male physician deaths, 1969-73	AMA age-adjusted	Actual/expected ♂ deaths=0.747 Actual/expected deaths=0.841		Medical= surgical specialty. General practitioners higher	Specific causes of death not investigated	
Sakinofsky I	England and Wales physicians 1970-72	Census data	♂ physician rate 3x greater than ♂ population; Single ♀ physician rate 2.5x greater than ♀ population	N.A. ♂ 14 ♀			Partially age adjusted

TABLE 6-1 (Continued)

Author	Basic Population and Year	Method	Suicide Rate	# of Suicides	Suicide Preference	Comment	Methodologic Comments
Watterson DJ	British Columbia physicians, 1970-74	Surveyed psychiatrists	Physicians 36.5/100,000	7 ♂ 0 ♀	Highest in ophthalmology & psychiatry	No relationship to sex or age	Survey of psychiatrists may well underestimate rate; no relationship to age is very unusual; low number of cases
Pepitone-Arreola Rockwell F, et al	U.S. medical students	Surveyed medical schools	15.6/100,000 ♂ 18.9/100,000 ♀	34 ♂ 9 ♀		Similar to population rate for age for ♂ 3 x higher for ♀ medical students than female population	Survey
Revicki DA, May HJ	North Carolina 1978-82	Death certificates	Physicians Others 31/100,000	13 ♂		Physician rate less than pharmacists, higher than dentists and nurses; 2/3 physician suicides 65 years or older; 85% depressed	Age adjusted

the professional rate of 55/100,000. The number of female physician suicides was too small to generalize an overall female physician suicide rate, but the female health care professional rate for suicide was 33/100,000/year compared to other professional-technical fields of 19/100,000/year. In addition, the data is rather old at this point, and there are few newer studies. The remainder of the studies show substantial disparity in the rate of suicide; however, it would appear that the male physician suicide rate is somewhere between 30-40/100,000 and the female physician suicide rate may be close to it.

The American Medical Association and the American Psychiatric Association recently completed a study of physician suicide (Council on Scientific Affairs). In this study, in-depth interviews with individuals close to physicians who died, primarily between 1982 and 1984, were conducted. There were 142 deaths by suicide and 101 deaths from other causes, which were matched by sex and age. Those who committed suicide differed from the controls: more chronic mental disorder, suicide attempts or verbalizations, mental health treatment, drug problems, psychiatric hospitalization, self-prescription of psycho-active drug, alcohol-related social problems, losses (personal, professional or financial), violence toward spouse, and alcohol or mental illness in family of origin. However, only four factors remained in multivariate analysis: prior suicide attempt, suicidal verbalizations, self-prescribed psychoactive drugs and financial losses. Of note, 65% of the suicides were successful on the first try.

Mortality series (1925 [Emerson], 1938-42 [Dublin], 1949-51 [Dickinson], 1969-73 [Goodman], 1970-72 [Sakinofsky] and one cohort study [Williams] have found physicians to have a lower mortality rate than the public. Their individual causes of death varied somewhat, but the relatively consistent findings were increased deaths from heart disease and suicide, and lower deaths from accidents. The studies of Emerson, Dublin, Dickinson and Goodman compared AMA data to national statistics. The three early studies were generally considered to be only males (there were not many female physicians); but the 1969-73 study (Goodman) found that male physicians had an actual/expected death rate of 74.7%; female physicians 84.1%. Bruce (1965) also found that anesthesiologists died less frequently from accidents than did the general population.

In summary, male physicians have had a slightly lower death rate than the public, but have been found consistently to have a higher suicide rate. A variety of methodologies have come to the same conclusion. No specialty preference can be determined, although several studies have suggested that psychiatrists and ear/nose/throat physicians are particularly at risk. Female physician suicides have not been studied little, and no series had a large enough number from which to generalize. It would also appear that female physician suicides are higher than the general female population, but perhaps about equivalent to their male physician counterparts.

Two additional points need to be made. First, there are many ways to commit suicide. In general, physicians use drugs more frequently than other people in committing suicide (Rose 1973, Craig, Blachly, Pitts, Steppacher, DeSole, Revicki). Many so-called 'accidents,' such as one-car accidents, may be hidden suicides. Physicians, however, have a lower mortality rate from accidents than the general population. Perhaps they are less frequently in situations where accidental death can occur. Or, perhaps some of the apparently high suicide rate is actually not what it appears--maybe some of the so-called higher rate of accidents in the general population are actually suicides. Physicians may just use handier means--drugs--more often than the violence of accidents, thereby being identified more readily as suicide victims.

A second point in the literature concerns female physician suicides. At least two of the papers (which share one author) reporting on female physician suicides note that the high incidence may be indicative of a high incidence of affective disorders and depression (Craig, Pitts). This is particularly interesting since the rates of suicide they found in both series for female physicians (40.5/100,000 [Craig] and 40.7/100,000 [Pitts]) were very similar to those for male physicians in each of their studies (38.3/100,000 [Craig] and 39.1/100,000 [Pitts]), and less than that for male physicians in other series (79/100,000 [Rose 1973] and 14/1337 [Thomas]). The same authors do not, however, indicate that male physicians should be similarly investigated for affective disorders. Such psychological studies of female physicians have been attempted and will be discussed in the next section on mental illness. The authors' conclusion of high rates of affective disorders only for female physicians raises the question of bias.

However, it is not clear why women physicians should have a rate of suicide substantially higher than other women, with only a small difference between men physicians and other men. The similar rates for men and women physicians could mean that it is primarily a result of the stresses or particular aspects of the profession that leads to suicide. Another possibility is that women physicians have a higher rate of suicide completion per attempt (Carlson and Miller) than other women, as they have more effective information on which to decide their suicide method. (We do not have figures on the rate of suicide attempts versus completed suicide for women physicians to verify or refute this possibility.) Perhaps women who enter medicine are different in premorbid characteristics than other women, or that factors that predispose to successful entry into medical school also predispose toward suicide. Alternatively, women physicians have greater stress in comparison to other women than men physicians to other men.

It is Generally Believed that Physicians Have a Greater Incidence of Drug and Alcohol Abuse than the General Public, Although There is Minimal Data to Support this Contention. When Addiction Occurs, it is More Likely to be to Available Alcohol or Prescription Drugs. There is Insufficient Evidence to State that Physicians Have a Greater Incidence of Other Mental Illnesses, nor that Female Physicians Have High Rates of Drug or Alcohol Abuse.

Methodologic problems also plague the data on mental illness and drug and alcohol abuse among physicians. There is a general belief that physicians have a greater incidence of drug abuse than the general public, and this belief seems to be self-perpetuating in the literature. One author references another author who references another author or just states that physicians have high rates of drug abuse. There is not a single well-controlled study with sufficient numbers of physicians to indicate true inferential statistics. This seems to be an instance where inherent belief has substantially biased studies and their conclusions, which has then continued unchallenged in the literature, a well-known phenomenon (Nisbett). When there are studies that one could reasonably trust, they only look at one aspect of addiction. But drug and alcohol abuse are related, similar problems. To truly compare the rates of abuse among physicians to those of the public, one must consider all drug and alcohol abuse, not just drug or alcohol, or just one drug.

In considering the studies, one must also consider the bias that may exist in mechanisms that detect the physician addict. Physicians may be more likely to be detected because of prescription monitoring systems in the United States and because of their proximity to other individuals, i.e., other health care professionals, who can identify addiction and who have a reason to report the individual and thus prevent harm to patients. On the other hand, physicians may be unwilling to report fellow physicians. Which way this bias operates in unclear.

Overall, there are serious problems with the studies of physician alcohol and drug abuse. This is not to say that physicians cannot be said to have 'high' rates of alcohol or drug abuse--anything above zero can be too 'high;' however, it makes it difficult to say that physicians are uniquely susceptible. A similar point is made by Brewster (1986), who also believes that "physicians may not be unusually likely to have such problems."

TABLE 6-2 Physician Psychiatric Morbidity Studies

Author	Basic Population	Year	Method of Study	Rate	Specialty Preference	Comments	Methodologic Problems
Modlin HC,	65 narcotic addicts presented to Meninger Foundation	15 year period prior to 1964	Personal knowledge + charts	46% physicians # = 30 2 suicides		5 left against medical advice	Psychiatric practice experience may be skewed
Pearson MM, et al	Psychiatric admissions to two Philadelphia hospitals	15 year period prior to	Personal knowledge + charts 1960	13/2441 one admissions = 5.7% physicians; over 15 years 71 patients = 3% of private patients 13.6% female		27% addicted 42% recovered or much improved	Psychiatric hospital experience may be skewed
Putnam PL, et al	68 male physician narcotic addicts admitted to USPHS Hospital; controls from AMA directory	1952-1962		80/2999 discharged were physicians = 2.7%	No specialty preference	3 were alcoholics	Criteria for entry to USPHS Hospital not specified. Hospital experience may be skewed

TABLE 6-2 (Continued)

Author	Basic Population	Year	Method of Study	Rate	Preference	Specialty Comments	Methodologic Problems
a'Brook MF, et al	Northampton, England 192 physicians at 2 inpatient facilities + 1 outpatient psychiatry practice; 2 control groups 1. new physician in Medical Register 2. matched patients at same sights	1954-1964	Personal knowledge + charts	9% ♀	Psychiatrists over-represented in out-patients	More physicians had drug addiction than controls, no difference alcoholism	Psychiatric hospitals and out-patient practices may be skewed
Duffy JC, et al	93 physician psychiatric patients at Mayo Clinic	1956-1963	Personal knowledge + charts		No specialty preference	47 alcohol or drug addiction or both; 21 left against medical advice	Psychiatric practice experience may be skewed
Vincent MO, et al	93 physician patients admitted to private psychiatric hospital	1960-67	Personal knowledge + charts	6.5% ♀	Psychiatric anesthesiologists	30% alcohol abuse 27% drug abuse; many signed out against medical advice	Psychiatric hospital experience may be skewed

TABLE 6-2 (Continued)

Author	Basic Population	Year	Method of Study	Rate	Preference	Specialty Comments	Methodologic Problems
Vincent MO,	167 physicians admitted to private psychiatric hospital, Ontario	1960-74		7.8% of physicians admitted were female		Female under represented	Psychiatric hospital experience may be skewed
Murray RM	36 male physician patients; 5 female physician patients at London Hospital	1964-73	Charts and follow-up	12.2% ♂		56.1% also abused drugs; 4 certain or probable suicides at follow-up; only 9 "practicing satisfactorily"	Local hospital experience may be skewed; low number of cases
Watterson DJ	British Columbia physicians	1970-74	Survey of psychiatrists problems	1.27% per year had psychiatric			Psychiatric practices may be skewed
Russell AT, et al	3737 psychiatric residents	July 1971-June 1972	Questionnaire to program directors	Suicide rate 106/100,000; 7.7% had serious psychiatric difficulties in residency program			Survey of program directors may underestimate psychiatric morbidity; small numbers of of suicides

TABLE 6-2 (Continued)

Author	Basic Population	Year	Method of Study	Rate	Preference	Specialty Comments	Methodologic Problems
Valko RJ, et al	53 who just completed internships in St. Louis	1972	Structured interview; Feighner criteria for depression	30% depressed during internship		"No drug or alcoholic use"	Small numbers
Valliant GE, et al	47 physicians part of follow-up study of college sophmores) 79 socioeconomically matched controls	Around 1972	questionnaire or interviews	Physicians ↑ poor marriages, ↑ drug and alcohol abuse ↑ psychotherapy			Small numbers
Bissell L, et al	98 recovered male alcoholic physicians members of AA	1975-1976	50-part questionnaire		Psychiatrists over-represented 22% did not seek help other then from AA	53% consulted psychiatrist,	Subjects identified through AA
Clayton PJ, et al	111 female white physicians in St. Louis area; 103 control female white Ph.D.'s	Around 1980	Personal interview Feighner criteria for affective disorder		39% ♀ physician affective disorder 30% ♀ psychologist affective disorder	No excess of psychiatrists	Appears to be same population as #41

TABLE 6-2 (Continued)

Author	Basic Population	Year	Method of Study	Rate	Preference	Specialty Comments	Methodologic Problems
Welner A, et al	111 female white physicians in St. Louis area; 103 control female white Ph.D.'s	Around 1980	Personal inter view Feighner criteria for affective disorder	51% ♀ physicians affective disorder 32% ♀ psychologists affective disorder	Psychiatrists over-represented		Appears to be same pop-ulation as #42
Zoccolillo M, et al	304 1st and 2nd year medical students; 79% response rate	1982-84	Beck Depression Inventory and Diagnostic Interview Schedule	12% major depression N=35	N.A.	N=10 had other psychiatric disorder as well. Higher rate of depression than general public for students before and during medical school	
Niven RG, et al	399 physicians at a continuing education meeting in Minnesota; mostly family physicians; 80% response rate	Around 1983	Self-administered alcoholism screening test	5% possible alcoholics 2% probable alcoholics	N.A.	Similar rate to general population given same instrument	Self-report

TABLE 6-2 (Continued)

Author	Basic Population	Year	Method of Study	Rate	Preference	Specialty Comments	Methodologic Problems
McAuliffe WE, et al	500 physicians 504 medical students 510 pharmacists 470 pharmacy students New England	1984	Surveys of drug use	25% physicians treated themselves with psychoactive drug, 10% use drugs recreationally 3% drug dependance. This was higher rates than pharmacists.	Psychiatrists had higher rates of drug use.	Recreational use similar to several other types of groups in society	Self-report
Maddux JF, et al	133 senior medical students; 69% response rate	1984	Survey	11% substance abuse symptoms (N=14, 6 from cigarettes) 25% used illicit substances in previous year	N.A.	Use of drugs associated with depressed mood	Self-report
Reuben	68 medical residents at Rhode Island Hospital	1985	Center for Epidemiological Studies Depression Scale	21.4% depression symptoms. First year residents 28.7%; third year residents 10.3%		Similar overall rate to population	

TABLE 6-2 (Continued)

Author	Basic Population	Year	Method of Study	Rate	Specialty Preference	Comments	Methodologic Problems
Clark DC, et al 1987	116 first year medical students with fewer on follow-up surveys	About 1982-86	Surveys of alcohol use; Research Diagnostic Criteria	11% excessive drinking 18% alcohol abusers sometime during medical school; 22% of σ, 10% of φ abused alcohol	N.A.		Self-report
Clark DC Zeldow PB	121 medical students mid-western school	? 1982-86	Beck Depression Inventory	At least 12% depressed at any measuring point. σ and φ similar	N.A.	Scores increased peak at end of second year	
Baldwin DC, Jr, et al	2,046 senior medical students at 23 medical schools; 64% response rate	1987	Survey	Medical students had lower rate of use of cigarettes marijuana and elicit drugs than young adults or college students. 1.6% thought they needed help for abuse	N.A.		Self-report

Several studies are summarized in Table 6-2. Several are based on psychiatric hospitalizations or practices, a method that makes generalization very difficult because of pre-selection of individuals. Vincent (1969) found females underrepresented; a'Brook (1967) and Pearson (1960) found them overrepresented. Drug and alcohol abuse was found to be prevalent by Duffy (1964) and Valliant (1970). Drug abuse was prevalent in the physician series of Modlin (1964), Pearson (1960), and a'Brook (1967). At least one study (Putnam) found a low rate of alcoholism among physician narcotic addicts (3/68 male physicians), and Pond (1969) believed there was no difference in drug or alcohol abuse compared to the general public based on his private practice experience. Morse (1984) found that physicians treated for alcoholism or drug dependence had a better prognosis.

Another study method is the use of surveys. There are several recent surveys of medical students (Conard, Clark, Maddux, Balwin). Conard (1988) surveyed fourth year medical students at 13 medical schools. The return rate was a low 41%; in the previous month, 88% used alcohol, 17% marijuana, 6% cocaine, 2% tranquilizers and 1% amphetamines. These rates of use were lower than age and sex cohorts, with the exception of opiates, where use was same, and tranquilizers/alcohol, where use was higher. Another recent survey of one medical school class, completed in longitudinal fashion (Clark 1987), found that 11% of the students met criteria for excessive drinking for at least one 6-month period. Women drank substantially less than the men; 22% of the men abused alcohol, but only 10% of the women did. Maddux (1986) also offers data on medical student drug use, and about 25% of the senior medical students had used illicit drugs in the previous year. Baldwin et al, looking at survey data from 23 medical schools in 1987, found rates of use of cigarettes and marijuana and other illicit substances to be substantially less than among other young adults or college students.

McAuliffe (1986) surveyed medical students and practicing physicians. In the previous year, a quarter of the physicians had treated themselves with a psychoactive drug, and an additional 10% used a recreational drug. 10% of the physicians reported regular, current drug use that was not prescribed by another physician; 3% had a history of drug dependence. Practicing physicians were more likely to treat themselves with drugs than to use them recreationally. The use was higher for physicians than for surveyed pharmacists and higher for medical students than for pharmacy students, but the rate of self-reported drug dependence was not. Use was higher among younger respondents. As noted by the authors, the overall rates of recreational use of drugs by the physicians and medical students was similar to other groups cited in the literature.

Yet others seem to assume that alcoholism or drug abuse is a particular problem for physicians without specific evidence (Fox, Bissell, Glatt, Scheiber, Murray). The specialty of psychiatry was overrepresented in two studies of drug and alcohol abuse (a'Brook, Bissell). Psychiatry residency directors (Russell) reported that 7.7% of psychiatry residents had serious problems during their graduate training and that there were 4 suicides (a high rate of 106/100,000).

State boards of medical examiners are another source of information. In 11 years, Arizona noted 1.7% of their physicians came before the board for disciplinary action for drug dependence; Connecticut had 0.9% in 6 years, and Oregon had 2.0% in 10 years (AMA Council on Mental Health). The similar figures for alcoholism were 3.2% in Arizona and 2.3% in Oregon. Garb (1965) surveyed state boards and found that from January 1960 to December 1964, 235 of 95,257 physicians (equivalent to 247/100,000 or 0.2%) in 20 states (those with adequate reporting mechanisms) were reported for meperidine addiction. However, it would appear that alcohol or other substance abuse are the most common reasons for physicians to have difficulties with their licenses (Shore).

Physicians may have a slightly different pattern of addiction from the population at large. They tend not to be street drug addicts and may have different socioeconomic characteristics. In the older literature (Modlin, Garb, Rasor), when they are addicted, physicians seem to be more likely to be addicted to meperidine, although as previously stated, the data on which this assumption is based has significant problems. A continuing trend is suggested by the study of Baldwin (1988) with medical students using only alcohol and tranquilizers but using other drugs less than other young adults or college students.

Physicians have Other Psychiatric Problems, Particularly Depression During the Training Years. Female Medical Students are More Likely to Seek Psychological Services. Some have Suggested that Women Physicians have a Higher Incidence of Affective Disorders than Men Physicians.

In spite of methodologic problems in the studies, one recurring theme is that physician psychiatric patients appear to be difficult patients--to have a high level of denial and frequently to sign out of the hospital setting against medical advice (Vincent 1976, a'Brook, Duffy, Modlin). Stoudemire (1983) believes that there is significant denial among physicians of their personal problems as well as denial of other physicians' problems, sometimes leading to suboptimal care.

Davidson (1978), Ghadirian (1982), Lloyd and Gartrell (1981), Heins (1979) and Lloyd (1983) have reported that women medical students seek psychiatric help substantially more frequently than men students. Of students seeking psychiatric help (Lloyd 1983) at one medical school, the women reported more depression and greater overall symptomatology, but there was no significant difference in primary diagnosis. About 40% of the complaints were primarily about problems other than those related to the pressures of medical school. Men were more likely to have a secondary diagnosis of obsessive-compulsive personality disorder and depression. In Ghardirian's study, 12.7% of students said in a survey that they had sought psychiatric help. Clark (1988) found that women medical students had similar neuroticism scores to men for the first three years of medical school, but in the fourth year, the men's scores dropped, suggesting the women were more anxious in the fourth year. There were no differences in perceived stress between the women and men. It may be that women and men have similar levels of stress and psychologic symptoms but women are more likely to seek help.

Depression is clearly common during the training years. Clark (1988) found that men and women had similar scores for the Beck Depression Inventory during medical school, and that at least 12% had BDI scores >14 (>20 almost always indicates a major depression) at any assessment during the first three years of medical school. Similarly, Zoccolillo (1986) found a rate of depression (by the Beck Depression Inventory and Diagnostic Interview Schedule) of 12% during the first two years of medical school, a rate three times the general population, and that more medical students had a history of depression prior to coming to medical school than was true of the general population in other studies. The rate of depression was similar for the men and women.

Residents also have psychological difficulties. More women (64%) than men (51.7%) family practice residents said they had had experienced personal, emotional, behavioral or mental problems than concerned them in the preceding year (Young). 17% of the women and 10% of the men considered their problems significant enough to seek professional help. Another study of family practice residents (Lemkau) found that they scored moderately high on measures of burnout, with no differences between the men and women. 30% of residents just completing internships in various specialties reported a depression had occurred during their internship, using the Feighner criteria (Valko 1975). 38% of the depressed residents considered quitting medicine. Many had previous psychiatric problems or family histories of psychiatric illness. A similar rate of depression (27% of 55) was reported among interns in their first six months by Clark (1984) using the Schedule for Affective Disorders and Schizophrenia-Lifetime

Version (SADS-L) and the Beck Depression Inventory. Reuben (1985) found a 29% prevalence rate of depression in 68 first-year medicine residents using the Center for Epidemiological Studies Depression Scale. The overall rate for all medicine residents was similar to the population. No comment was made on the rate by sex.

Two studies that purport to study the incidence of affective disorders in female physicians highlight a problem of medical literature that may not be uncommon, but complicates this look at the mental health of female physicians. The two studies (Welner, Clayton) share four authors, apparently have the same population base, controls and interview data, yet reach significantly different conclusions. One hundred eleven female physicians and 103 control female Ph.D.s were interviewed in the St. Louis area. The Feighner criteria, later criticized thoroughly (Stevens), were used to determine the presence or absence of affective disorders. Welner (1979) concluded that 51% of the female physicians and 32% of the female Ph.D.'s had affective disorders; Clayton et al (1980) concluded that the figures were 39% and 30%. Welner concluded that psychiatrists were overrepresented in the affective disorder group; Clayton said they were not. Either way, the incidence would appear to be high, but the differences, along with the questions concerning the criteria utilized to determine the presence of affective disorder, call both studies into question. These studies and the potential methodologic problems are also discussed by Carlson and Miller (1981).

Of note, depression is more common in women than men in the general population (Robins). Thus, a greater incidence of depression in women physicians than men would not be unexpected. In fact, Zoccolillo (1988) believes that the increase in depression for men physicians is greater in relationship to the general public (15% compared to 1%), which is also suggested by the studies which found similar rates of depression for men and women during medical school or residency. Also, when considering the substantial relationship between depression and suicide, the rate of depression is so high that the rate of suicide begins to look low!

Male and Female Physicians have a Lower than Average Divorce Rate Compared to Other Employed or Professional Individuals, Although the Divorce Rate is Twice as High for Female Physicians as for Male Physicians. Almost Half of Married Female Physicians have Physician Spouses.

"Most people look upon marriage as a potential support to male physicians, but see marriage as a potential burden for most female physicians."

(Vincent) Fifteen percent of applicants to medical school are married, and two percent are either widowed, separated or divorced (Gordon). Two surveys of practicing physicians, one of Medical Economics readers (Kirchner), and one of randomly selected physicians in Ramsey County, Minnesota (Garvey), found the divorce rate lower than the general population. The Medical Economics survey (Kirchner) found 7% re-married, 3% divorced, and 1% separated, although female physicians were more likely to be divorced (figures for female physicians were not pro- vided); 8.8% of the Ramsey County physicians were divorced at some time--both lower rates than the general population. The Ramsey County survey (Garvey) and another study (Valliant) found that longer hours were not related to more divorces, however, these were studies of male, not female, physicians.

Although only 1/5 and 1/3 of women physicians married in the latter half of the nineteenth century, more recent surveys indicate that about three-quarters get married (80% 1976 [Cohen], 77% 1977 [Heins], 78% 1970 [Westling-Wikstrand], 75% 1980 [Ordway], 72% 1972 [Standley], 77% 1969 [Powers], 69% 1953 [Dykman]). Generally, about half were married to physicians. Interestingly, one of these authors (Westling-Wikstrand) also found reported stress and anxiety to be higher in the female physicians who married early than in those who were not married or married later; and that married physicians, especially those who married early, had less successful careers.

There are few figures on divorce for women physician. One author reporting from a Medical Economics survey (Kirchner), says divorce is higher for women than for men in her survey, but does not provide figures. In a study of marital stability among physicians in California in 1968 (Rose 1972), female physicians had a divorce rate of 23.9/100,000/year compared to the female population rate of 22.6/100,000/year. The corresponding rate for male physicians was only 16.0/100,000/year. Doherty and Burge (1989), using 1980 Census figures, report that the divorce rate for women physicians was 82/1,000, compared to 106/1,000 for employed women and 93/1,000 for other professional women. The same figures for men were 43/1,000, 55/1000 and 55/1,000, respectively.

Perhaps the quote is right. Marriage may be more of a burden for the female physician than the male physician because she has more of the household responsibilities (Heins, Research Committee of AMWA). Therefore female physicians get divorced more frequently or do less well in their careers. At least two other reasons could be postulated for these statistics--men have more difficulty accepting a career-oriented wife, as has been the sociological inbreeding, or, perhaps, female physicians, being socioeconomically and mentally independent, have less reason to remain in a bad or unsatisfying marriage, and therefore get out, i.e, get divorced.

Summary and Discussion

McCue (1982) summarizes stress for physicians in the following way: "I believe that the stresses of medical practice result from one or more of the following situations peculiar to medicine: working with intensely emotional aspects of life governed by strong cultural codes for behavior, e.g., suffering, fear, sexuality, and death; inadequate training for fundamental professional tasks, e.g., handling "problem" patients; and demands from society or patients that cannot be reasonably met, e.g., the need for certainty when current medical knowledge allows only approximation." Another author (Cartwright) notes, "The pressures of training and practice, the number of patients seen, the psychological drain associated with assuming responsibility for others' lives, the affective climate surrounding disease, as well as contradictory and unrealizable aspects of current roles of healers, are among the more obvious factors implicated in the search for sources of distress."

The sources of stresses in medical practice appear to be changing over time, with more stress now from malpractice litigation, having to give up certain aspects of medical work, threats of physical harm, and peer review (Mawardi). Time pressures are recurrently mentioned (Cartwright, Mawardi, Spears). A pressure that may already be present to a certain degree, and bound to increase in the future, is the competition among the increasing number of physicians and nonphysician health care practitioners, the same pressure that was blamed for the high suicide rate among physicians at the turn of the century (Anonymous). Certainly there are significant sources of stress for today's physician.

Physicians also have the opportunity to provide help to many, an altruism that permeates practice, however invisible at times. Whether the stressors outweigh the benefit of altruism, along with the benefits of fairly high prestige and socioeconomic standing, is an individual matter, but one that should be the interest of all physicians. With relatively high suicide rates and higher divorce rates among female physicians, there is evidence that at least some physicians feel the pressure. While stress is not the only reason for physician impairment, there is opportunity to positively change its potential impact. All physicians should take cognizance of their own stress levels, and all should practice preventive medicine for themselves. More on this in later chapters!

References

Abram RJ, Ed. Send us a lady physician: Women doctors in America 1835-1920. W.W. Norton & Company, New York, 1985.

a'Brook MF, Hailston JD, McLauchlan IEJ. Psychiatric illness in the medical profession. Br J Psychiatry 1967;113:1013-1023.

AMA Council on Mental Health. The sick physician -- Impairment by psychiatric disorders, including alcoholism and drug dependence. JAMA 1973;223(6): 684-687.

Andrews JG, Tennant C. Life events and psychological illness. Psychological Medicine 1978;8:545-549.

Annotated Bibliography of Cause-of-Death Validation Studies: 1958-1980. Data evaluation and methods research series 2, No. 89, U.S. Department of Health and Human Services, Public Health Service, Office of Health Research, Statistics, and Technology, National Center for Health Statistics, DHHS Publication No. (PHS) 82-1361, 1982.

Anonymous. Suicide of physicians and the reasons. JAMA 1903;41:263-264.

Baldwin DC, Jr., Conard S, Hughes H, Achenbach KE, Sheehan DV. Substance use and abuse among senior medical students in 23 medical schools. Research in Medical Education, 1988 Proceedings of the Twenty-Seventh Annual Conference, Association of American Medical Colleges, Washington, DC, 1988.

Bissell L, Jones RW. The alcoholic physician: A survey. Am J Psych 1976;133(10): 1142-1146.

Blachly PH, Disher W, Roduner G. Suicide by physicians. Bull Suicidology Dec 1968:1-18.

Blachly PH, Osterud HT, Josslin R. Suicide in professional groups. N Engl J Med 1963;268(230):1278-1282.

Brewster JM. Prevalence of alcohol and other drug problems among physicians. JAMA 1986;255(14):1913-1920.

Bruce DL, Eide KA, Linde HW, Eckenhoff JE. Causes of death among anesthesiologists: A 20-year survey. Anesthesiology 1965;29:565-569.

Carlson GA, Miller DC. Suicide, affective disorder, and women physicians. Am J Psychiatry 1981;138(10):1330-1335.

Cartwright LK. Sources and effects of stress in health careers. In Health Psychology. Ed. by Stone GC, Gohen F, Adler NE, et al. Jossey-Bass, 1979.

Clark DC, Eckenfeis EJ, Daugherty SR, Fawcett J. Alcohol-use patterns through medical school: A longitudinal study of one class. JAMA 1987;257(21): 2921-2926.

Clark DC, Salazar-Gruesco E, Grabler P, Fawcett J. Predictors of depression during the first 6 months of internship. Am J Psychiatry 1984;141:1095-1098.

Clark DC, Zeldow PB. Vicissitudes of depressed mood during four years of medical school. JAMA 1988;260(17):2521-2528.

Clayton PJ, Marten S, Davis MA, Wochnik E. Mood disorders in women professionals. J Affective Disorders 1980;2:37-46.

Cohen ED, Korper SP. Women in medicine: A survey of professional activities, career interruptions, and conflict resolutions -- Trends in medical education and specialization. First of Two Parts. Conn Med 1976;40(2):103-110.

Conard S, Hughes P, Baldwin DC, Achenbach KE, Sheehan DV. Substance use by fourth-year students at 13 U.S. medical schools. J Med Educ 1988;63:747-758.

Cook DJ, Hole DJ. The aetiological importance of stressful life events. Br J Psychiatry 1983;143:397-400.

Council on Scientific Affairs. Results and implications of the AMA-APA physician mortality project: Stage II. JAMA 1987;257(21):2949-2953.

Craig AG, Pitts FN, Jr. Suicide by physicians. Dis Nerv System 1968;29:763-772.

Davidson VM. Coping styles of women medical students. J Med Educ 1978;53: 902-907.

DeSole DE, Singer P, Aronson S. Suicide and role strain among physicians. Int J Soc Psychiatry 1969;15:294-301.

Dickinson FG, Martin LW. Physician mortality, 1949-51. JAMA 1956;162(16): 1088-1093.

Doherty WJ, Burge SK. Divorce among physicians: Comparisons with other occupational groups. JAMA 1989;261(16):2374-2377.

Doll R, Peto R. Mortality in relation to smoking: 20 years' observation on male British doctors. Br Med J 1976;2:1525-1536.

Doll R, Peto R. Mortality among doctors in different occupations. Br Med J 1977;1:1433-1436.

Dublin L, Spiegelman M. The longevity and mortality of American physicians, 1938-1942. JAMA 1947;134(15):1211-1215.

Duffy JC, Litin EM. Psychiatric morbidity of physicians. JAMA 1964;189(13): 989-992.

Dykman RA, Stalnaker J. Survey of women physicians graduating from medical school 1925-1940. J Med Educ 1957;32:3-38.

Emerson H, Hughes HE. Death rates of male white physicians in the United States, by age and cause. Am J Public Health 1926;16:1088-1093.

Fox JD. Narcotic addiction among physicians. J Mich Med Soc February 1957: 214-217, 226.

Garb S. Narcotic addiction in nurses and doctors. Nurs Outlook 1965;13:30-34.

Garvey M, Tuason V. Physician marriages. J Clin Psychiatry 1979;l40:129-131.

Ghadirian AM, Engelsmann F. Emotional disorders among medical students. J Psychiatric Treatment and Evaluation 1982;4:459-461.

Glatt MM. Alcoholism and drug dependence in doctors and nurses. Br Med J 1968;1:380-381.

Goodman LJ. The longevity and mortality of American physicians, 1969-1973. Milbank Mem Fund Q 1975;53:353-375.

Gordon TL, Johnson DG. Study of U.S. medical school applicants, 1976-1977. J Med Educ 1978;53:873-897.

Heins M, Smock S, Martindale L, Jacobs J, Stein M. Comparison of the productivity of women and men physicians. JAMA 1977;237(23):2514-2517.

Heins M, Thomas J. Women medical students: A new appraisal. J Am Med Wom Assoc 1979;34:408-415.

Kirchner M. After hours. Med Econ October 1, 1979:9-32.

Lemkau JP, Purdy RR, Rafferty JP, Rudisill JR. Correlates of burnout among family practice residents. J Med Educ 1988;63:682-691.

Lloyd C. Sex differences in medical students requesting psychiatric intervention. J Nerv & Ment Disease 1983;171(9):535-545.

Lloyd C, Gartrell NK. Sex differences in medical student mental health. Am J Psychiatry 1981;138:1346-1351.

Maddux JF, Hoppe SK, Costello RM. Psychoactive substance use among medical students. Am J Psychiatry 1986;143(2):187-191.

Mawardi BH. Satisfactions, dissatisfactions, and causes of stress in medical practice. JAMA 1979;241(14):1483-1486.

McAuliffe WE, Rohman M, Santangelo S, Feldman B, Magnuson E, Sobol A, Weissman J. Psychoactive drug use among practicing physicians and medical students. N Engl J Med 1986;315(13):805-810.

McCue JD. The effects of stress on physicians and their medical practice. N Engl J Med 1982;306(8):458-476.

Modlin HC, Montes A. Narcotic addiction in physicians. Am J Psych 1964;121: 358-365.

Morse RM, Martin MA, Swenson WM, Niven RG. Prognosis of physicians treated for alcoholism and drug dependence. JAMA 1984;251(6):743-746.

Murray RM. Characteristics and prognosis of alcoholic doctors. Br Med J 1976;2:1537-1539.

Nisbett R, Ross L. Human Inference: Strategies and shortcoming of social judgment. Prentice-Hall, New Jersey, Inc., 1980.

Niven RG, Hurt RD, Morse RM, Swenson WM. Alcoholism in physicians. Mayo Clin Proc 1984;59:12-16.

Ordway JE. Professional women's unanticipated contented feelings after the birth of a child. J Am Med Wom Assoc 1980;35(10);240-245.

Pearson MM, Strecker EA. Physicians as psychiatric patients: private practice experience. Am J Psych 1960;116:915-919.

Pepitone-Arreola-Rockwell F, Rockwell D, Core N. Fifty-two medical student suicides. Am J Psychiatry 1981;138(2):198-201.

Pitts FN, Jr., Schuller AR, Rich CL, Pitts AF. Suicide among U.S. women physicians, 1967-1972. Am J Psychiatry 1979:136(5):694-196.

Pollock DA, Boyle CA, DeStefano F, Moyer LA, Kirk ML. Underreporting of alcohol-related mortality on death certificates of young US Army veterans. JAMA 1987;258(3):345-348.

Pond DA. Doctors' mental health. NZ Med J 1969;69(442):131-135.

Powers L, Parmelle RD, Wiesenfelder H. Practice patterns of women and men physicians. J Med Educ 1969;44:481-491.

Putnam PL, Ellinwood EH, Jr. Narcotic addiction among physicians: A ten-year follow-up. Am J Psych 1966;122:745-748.

Rasor RW, Crecraft HJ. Addiction to Meperidine (Demerol) Hydrochloride. JAMA 1955;157:654-657.

Research Committee of AMWA. Results of a pilot survey of household help problems of women physicians in the U.S. J Am Med Wom Assoc 1972;27(6): 324-327.

Reuben DB. Depressive symptoms in medical house officers. Arch Intern Med 1985;145:286-288.

Revicki DA, May HJ. Physician suicide in North Carolina. S Med J 1985;78(10): 1205-1207.

Rich CL, Pitts FN, Jr. Suicide by psychiatrists: A study of medical specialists among 18,730 consecutive physician deaths during a five-year period, 1967-1972. J Clin Psychiatry 1980;41(8):261-263.

Robins LN, Helzer JE, Weissman MM, Orvaschel H, Gruenberg E, Burke JD, Regier DA. Lifetime prevalence of specific psychiatric disorders in three sites. Arch Gen Psychiatry 1984;41:949-958.

Rose KD, Rosow I. Marital stability among physicians. Cal Med, West J Med 1972;116(3):95-99.

Rose KD, Rosow I. Physicians who kill themselves. Arch Gen Psych 1973;29: 800-805.

Russell AT, Pasnau RA, Taintor ZC. Emotional problems of residents in psychiatry. Am J Psych 1975;132(3):263-267.

Sakinofsky I. Suicide in doctors and wives of doctors. Can Fam Physician 1980;26: 837-844.

Scheiber SC. Emotional problems of physicians: Nature and extent of problems. Ariz Med 1977;34(5):323-325.

Shore JH. The Oregon experience with impaired physicians on probation. JAMA 1987;257(21):2931-2934.

Smith SN, Blachly PH. Amphetamine usage by medical students. J Med Educ 1966; 41:167-170.

Spears BW. A time management system for preventing physician impairment. J Fam Pract 1980;13(1):75-80.

Standley K, Soule B. Women in professions: historic antecedents and current lifestyles. Presented at the American Psychological Association, Hawaii 1972.

Steppacher RC, Mausner JS. Suicide in male and female physicians. JAMA 1974;228(3):323-328.

Stevens JR, Shore J. Female physicians and primary affective disorder. Letter to the Editor. Arch Gen Psychiatry 1980;37:110-111.

Stoudemire A, Rhoads JM. When the doctor needs a doctor: Special considerations for the physician-patient. Ann Intern Med 1983;98(Part 1):654-659.

Thomas CB. Suicide among us: can we learn to prevent it? Hopkins Med J 1969;125(69):276-285.

Valko RJ, Clayton PJ. Depression in the internship. Dis Nerv Sys 1975;36:26-29.

Valliant GE, Sobowale NC, McArther C. Some psychological vulnerabilities of physicians. N Engl J Med 1972;287(8);372-375.

Vincent MO, Robinson EA, Latt L. Physicians as patients: private psychiatric hospital experience. Can Med Assoc J 1969;100(9):403-412.

Watkins C. Use of amphetamine by medical students. S Med J August 1970: 923-929.

Watterson DJ. Psychiatric illness in the medical profession: Incidence in relation to sex and field of practice. C Med Assoc J 1976;115:311-317.

Welner A, Marten S, Wochnick E, Davis MA, Rishman R, Clayton PJ. Psychiatric disorders among professional women. Arch Gen Psychiatry 1979;36:169-179.

Westling-Wikstrand H, Monk MA, Thomas CB. Some characteristics related to the career status of women physicians. Hopkins Med J 1970;127:273-286.

Williams SV, Munford RS, Colton T, Murphy DA, Poskanzer DC. Mortality among physicians: A cohort study. J Chronic Dis 1971;24:393-401.

Young EH. Relationship of residents' emotional problems, coping behaviors, and gender. J Med Educ 1987;62:642-650.

Zoccolillo M. Major depression during medical training. JAMA 1988;260:2560-2561.

Zoccolillo M, Murphy GE, Wetzel RD. Depression among medical students. J Affective Disorders 1986;11:91-96.

"Being a woman has been an advantage for me. Our society equates women with emotional sensitivity, so patients of both sexes feel freer to unburden themselves of feelings with me. Many of my women patients are sexual abuse victims who embrace work with a woman psychiatrist but remain distrustful of male psychiatrists. One of the greatest pleasures in my work is relieving the pain of these victims and teaching residents to be sensitive to their emotional needs."

Dr. Elizabeth Bowman
Academic Career - Psychiatrist
Married, no children, mid 30's

7
Women are Different:
Women Physicians' Way of Healing

Let's face it, women are different. There is a tremendous amount of sociological literature that shows how women are different from men. For example, women think differently (Belenky, Gilligan), have different bodies, conduct their lives differently, and have less position power. Differences between individual men and women may be more or less, but the groups as a whole show marked differences.

And, first and foremost, women physicians are women. Early sex-role orientations are highly reinforced (Williams and Best 1982, Weisman) and resistant to change (Weisman). Presuming that this means women physicians have more feminine characteristics than men physicians, how does being a woman influence how she practices the profession of medicine? Much of this book notes systematic differences between groups of men and women physicians. Certainly, many have suggested, from the last century (Walsh) to the present (Restak), that women can bring humanism and caring to the profession of medicine . At least one author (Restak) has gone so far as to declare that this is markedly positive for the patients: "We need more cheap, docile women doctors." What is the end result of the differences between men and women physicians? Are women physicians better healers than men physicians?

In general, there are no magic, firm answers. This chapter will attempt to use some of the 'softer' literature on women and women physicians to provide answers and speculate on possibilities.

Sex-Related Differences in Achievement

Women physicians are less successful than men physicians by classical definitions: they earn less money per hour, see fewer patients, have less academic success, and have less position power. In thinking about why this might be, there are four major theories: lower ability, less achievement-motivation or confidence, personality differences and discrimination.

Ability   Women and men physicians are similar in academic ability measured by traditional standards.

The evidence on ability reviewed in previous chapter indicates that women entering medical school are at least as qualified as men and do as well while in medical school.

There are those who think that men and women in the general population have differences in ability, such as with verbal or quantitative ability; however, the difference is about 1% of the variance for verbal and 4% for quantitative ability (Jacklin). A genetic hypothesis has not been confirmed for differences in quantitative ability through direct tests, possibly because of differential feedback given to girls and boys throughout school (Jacklin).

However, the literature on sex-related differences in ability is fraught with methodological issues. Jacklin (1981) identified ten major ones, including: problems with definition of 'difference'; confusion about statistically significant versus sufficient size effect; bias toward publishing studies showing differences; lack of control for differences in self-report by men and women (with men more defensive in self-reporting and less likely to disclose personal feelings); problems of within-sex versus between-sex differences; non-generalizable samples; and the large number of variables potentially confounded with sex. She notes that the better the sex-related research, the less sex has been found to account for variance in characteristics or behaviors. We believe her conclusions could be applied to sex-related differences between men and women physicians as well.

Overall, as Jacklin (1981) points out, a 20% difference between men and women may mean that 80% of the men and women are the same on any particular trait or behavior measured. This is often referred to as greater within-group than between-group variability. Similarly, it is likely that most men and women physicians are more comparable in ability than different.

Achievement Motivation and Confidence   Women physicians have less achievement-motivation, are less confident, less likely to choose risky situations, and face more anxiety over performance than men physicians. These characteristics are highly intertwined with personality (sex-role typing) differences and discrimination.

Men are believed to be more likely to attribute outcome to their ability, and consider their ability higher regardless of success or failure; women are believed to be more likely to attribute outcome to luck (Frieze). While meta-analysis of multiple studies confirmed these beliefs (Frieze), the differences were small and the author noted that some studies were contradictory. In one study not included in the meta-analysis, men attending local fairs were more likely to choose games requiring skill and to persist longer while women chose games involving luck (Deaux 1975), perhaps because of men's greater confidence in their own abilities.   In another study (Feather 1969), which looked at expectations, unexpected success was more attributed to luck and associated with greater satisfaction. The female subjects were lower in confidence and higher in inadequacy than male subjects and were more likely to attribute success or failure to luck.

Another way to consider confidence and achievement-motivation is to determine how men and women view other men's and women's abilities. Men are expected to be more successful (Feldman-Summers), and undergraduate subjects rated successful female physicians as more motivated than successful male physicians (Feldman-Summers). Male and female mental health therapists held similar concepts for healthy 'adults' and healthy men, but viewed healthy women as different than healthy adults (Broverman 1970).   When subjects were asked to rate the performance of males and females on male- or female-related tasks, subjects believed the males to be more skillful in either male- or female-related tasks, and the performance of the males to be more related to skill overall on the male-task (Deaux 1974).   In considering a male or female failing an exam for three sex-linked occupations (medicine, teaching and nursing), female subjects downgraded successful females in relationship to unsuccessful females but upgraded successful males in relationship to unsuccessful males regardless of the three occupations (Feather 1975). Overall, successful males and unsuccessful females were rated higher than either the unsuccessful males or successful females and males were given more credit for success and females more blame for failure.   Thus, attribution studies suggest that females should desire less success, as they will be blamed more for failure and receive less recognition for success.

Women are generally less confident in achievement settings, but this is probably dependent on the actual situation (Lenney). Women are more likely to be confident with 'feminine' tasks than 'masculine' tasks, even when the sex definitions have been manipulated (Lenney). Women are more likely to have more confidence when given clear feedback (Lenney). Lower confidence translates into choosing less demanding tasks and giving up more easily in the setting of failure (Lenney) and lower chances of success (Feather 1969).

Lower self-confidence is at least partially socially determined. Women are less confident in a social environment, but not when they work alone or do not expect their performance to be compared to others (Lenney). Hoffman (1972) agrees and argues that socialization encourages affiliation in young girls, and if achievement threatens affiliation, girls will sacrifice performance or experience anxiety. In other words, relationships are more important than achievement for women, leading to less self-confidence and less achievement motivation.

Women professional students also see themselves as more feminine than the ideal practitioner in their field (Giles, Davis, Coplin), and more so than men, speculatively leading to more anxiety about role performance.

The profession of medicine would appear to be a sex-linked area ('male') with high social interaction and unclear feedback on performance. Thus, the cited literature suggests that women physicians would: 1) be lower in confidence; 2) be less willing to choose high demand situations or those tasks considered 'masculine'; and 3) face more anxiety over their performance. At least partially as a result of these characteristics, they would be less successful.

In fact, the evidence in medicine, though limited in quantity and quality, suggests these hypotheses to be true. For example, women with mediocre performance in college are less likely to apply and, ultimately, get into medical school (Fiorentine). (This is similar to the fact that female high school students get better grades but are less likely to go on to college (Williams and Best).) Noncognitive variables are more predictive of women's performance in medical school whereas cognitive variables are predictive for men (Willoughby). Women are less likely to choose traditional male specialties or male tasks, and perform fewer risky procedures in practice (Ellsbury, Ogle). They feel less prepared for practice, particularly in surgical areas (Ellsbury). As noted in the Chapter on Mental Health, there is some evidence that women physicians face more anxiety or seek mental health care more frequently, at least during medical school. There is no literature on attributions for success of women physicians for themselves. On the other hand, at least one study suggests that the level of confidence of women physicians may improve from the time of entry to medical school to a follow-up 8 to 10 years later (Cartwright 1977). And, as seen already, women are less successful in medicine by traditional measurements.

Personality Differences Between Men and Women Physicians   Women physicians are more oriented to the doctor-patient relationship and the men physicians to techniques. Women physicians may also be more 'feminine' or 'androgynous'.
The major method of considering differences between men and women is sex-role typing. The Bem Sex-Role Inventory is a widely known instrument assessing traits frequently attributed to each sex. Masculine traits are described by such adjectives as aggressive, assertive, ambitious, competitive, dominant. Adjectives for feminine traits include compassionate,

understanding, sensitive to the needs of others, and yielding. In general, women score higher on feminine characteristics and men on masculine characteristics, with a third category being androgynous (high on both masculine and feminine behaviors), and the fourth being undifferentiated (low on both masculine and feminine behaviors) (Hoffman). Other terms are used to describe the differences: independent/instrumental/scientific/ reserved/technicalversusaffiliative/expressive/interpersonal/helping-oriented /humane. These sex stereotypes have changed very little in the United States over the last 16 years (Williams and Best 1990). The masculine profile tends to be valued more in our society (Broverman), probably because of higher levels of activity and strength in the definition (Best). Women do not see themselves as less 'good' (Williams and Best 1982), just less 'strong' and 'active' (Best).

It could be theorized that androgyny would be the best sex-role type for the physician, since the physician is expected to be independent and assertive yet responsive to the needs of others (Shapiro), i.e., a physician should combine the good aspects of both sexual stereotypes. The ideal physician is considered more androgynous than the ideal lawyer (compare Giles and Coplin). Medical students conceive of their ideal physician as androgynous (Giles); very similar findings held true for physician assistant students as well (Davis). Also, both male and female androgynous individuals, followed by masculine individuals, have more self-esteem and less neuroticism than feminine or undifferentiated individuals (Hoffman DM), another potential advantage of androgeny for physicians. Individuals tend to describe the ideal sex-role traits as at the androgynous level (Williams and Best 1982), and those who are androgynous are more flexible behaviorly, which would appear to have advantages for mental health (Williams and Best 1982). Consistent with this, Clark (1988) found that higher masculinity was associated with less depression for male medical students and women who were more aggressive, worldly, or not easily hurt had less depression. These differences in self-esteem and implied advantages for androgyny, however, do not clearly translate into differences in the health of the different sex-role types (Hoffman DM).

There is a little information available in the literature on the sex-role types of physicians. Williams and Best (1982) found women medical students to rate themselves as about the same femininity as typical female college students, but more feminine than the ideal physician (Giles). Since the ideal physician was androgynous, and male medical students rated themselves similarly androgynous, but female medical students rated themselves as farther from the ideal, i.e., more feminine (Giles), the female students could have more anxiety over their performance. Similarly, female physician assistant students (Davis) and law students (Coplin) rated themselves as more feminine than the ideal person in their profession. Shapiro (1983) found that female patients considered female physicians to be more androgynous, less masculine and more feminine than male physicians. There were no significant differences in the rating of the male and female physicians by male patients. Male medical students and male physicians saw female physicians as much more feminine and male physicians as much more masculine. Female medical students saw female physicians as more androgynous. Overall, women physicians were seen more as androgynous by patients and men physicians as undifferentiated. The authors conclude that male and female physicians are considered different from each other, but that the extent and type of differences are variable, depending upon who rated them.

Several studies, which have discussed various aspects of the personalities of men and women physicians using techniques other than traditional sex-role measures, in general confirm the sex-role typing of women physicians as possessing more feminine traits than men physicians. Several have found that women students are more attuned to patient relationships. For example, Cartwright (1972) found first- year women students had more sensitivity to relationships and more general acceptance of feelings than men students. Bergquist (1985) found women medical students placed more value on patient contact. Women medical student applicants (Roessler) scored higher on nurturing, change, impulsivity, understanding and harm avoidance and lower on dominance, exhibition and order scales. The accepted and rejected women medical students were not different. In a longitudinal survey, Leserman (1981) found new women students placed more value on psychosocial factors in health care. In an interesting twist on this question, Gross and Crovitz (1975) asked medical students to rate women medical students and women on different categories; the women medical students were rated as nurturant as women but more aggressive, exacting, enduring, achievement-oriented, intellectual and dominant than women in the general population.

With the Myers-Briggs Scale, Rezler & Buckley (1977) found that women medical students in general were guided more than other women health care professional students by thinking than feelings in their approach to work and other people. Unfortunately, they did not have comparison male students.

Within each group, there were marked differences among the students. In contrast, Maheux (1988) reported the professional and sociopolitical attitudes of 343 female and 380 male medical students from a northwestern state in 1979 to be similar, with increasing similarity at more advanced levels of training.

Crowson (1986) considered health locus of control of 21 men and 13 women internal medicine residents. This is a measure of the extent to which the individual perceives control of the results of his/her own behavior; for example, external locus of control suggests that luck explains what happens to individuals, whereas internal locus of control suggests that it is a result of internally controlled behavior. Crowson found the women had greater external locus of control ($p < 0.01$); however Frey (1981) had found no difference in a similar study of family practice first year residents. There have been no larger studies comparing locus of control nor elucidating the full implications of locus of control for physicians.

Lorber (1984) found that men and women practicing physicians similarly described the patients they liked best and least. Of the women and men physicians she interviewed, only one woman physician believed that women handled patients differently. However, when asked about their accomplishments in medicine, the women were more likely to discuss the personal or 'caring' aspect, and men therapeutic skills (Lorber 1984), consistent with typical sex-role typing. Women physicians may relate better to dying patients, finding it easier to discuss death and console families (Dickerson & Pearson).

Discrimination   Discrimination exists, but cannot solely account for the differences between men and women physicians.   Some patients prefer a specific sex of physician, dependent on the circumstances, the type of medical problem and expectations.
The evidence for discrimination is less palpable, but many women physicians believes it exists.   Just as sex-role stereotyping (a form of discrimination) has persisted--and there have been few public policy changes accompanying major changes in women's roles (Russo and Denmark)--discrimination based on sex exists, persists, and is likely to continue. A book has been devoted to discrimination faced by medical students, including multiple quotes and descriptions of the types of situations that occur (Campbell). Lorber (1984) believed that women physicians were discriminated against in practice, receiving fewer referrals from other physicians than men physicians because of discrimination.

Some patients may also discriminate, preferring not to see women physicians (Kasteler, Needle, Haar, Engleman).   Others prefer to see women physicians. Overall, women physicians have more women in their practices than do men physicians (Bowman, Challacombe, Hartzema); this is also true for patients with psychiatric problems (Fenton).   Earlier research in 1974 (Engleman) found that patients generally preferred male doctors and believed female doctors were less competent and experienced. Many believed they would not be willing to discuss certain things with women physicians. This negative attitude toward women physicians was particularly true for Spanish-speaking patients and far less true for obstetrics/gynecology patients and black women patients. Patients who had seen women physicians were more positive toward them.

Women patients may particularly prefer women physicians for specific types of exams, particularly those involving the breasts and pelvic organs. While this is probably true, it may only be true for a minority of women patients. Petravage (1979) found about 1/5 of her sample specifically preferred women physicians for breast and pelvic exams. In considering adolescents' anxiety before and after a pelvic examinations, Seymore (1986) found that those who had never had a pelvic examination before did better in a semi-erect position examined by a female physician, but those who had had pelvic examinations before did better in semi-erect position examined by a male physician. In another study (Philliber), female adolescent contraceptive patients also expressed desire for a female provider; this was more important to them than the ethnicity or age of the provider.

Ackerman-Ross (1980) similarly found that certain types of complaints predicted preference for same-sex physician, particularly sexual dysfunction followed by physical examination and blood in urine, with no difference by sex of the physician for sore throat. However, they found a general preference for same-sex physician, with men more strongly shifting to wanting male physicians for the more intimate problems than female patients to female physicians. Also, of importance to understanding this literature, patients were more likely to choose a physician of either sex who was more highly recommended by others. Thus, recommendation by others was more important than the sex of the physician in determining which physician the patient selected.

Patients may be more satisfied when they have the opportunity to choose their own physician, thus being able to choose one with the characteristics desired, whether or not one of the important aspects of choice is the sex of the physician. When not able to choose the physician, the patients may generally be less satisfied, particularly with physicians with non-normative characteristics, such as physicians who are women or black (Ross). For example, in the large group practices, patients were less satisfied with female doctors, Catholic doctors, and those from low status backgrounds, whereas this was not true in small practices.

Thus, there is selectivity on the part of patients for the sex of the physician, dependent on circumstances, the type of problem, and expectations. There is also discrimination within the medical field itself against women physicians. However, it is doubtful that discrimination is the full reason for the differences between men and women physicians.

The Evidence: Differences in Practice

There are some differences in practice styles between women and men physicians--in particular, women physicians spend more time with each patient. Quality of care appears to be the same and women and men physicians treat comparable patients similarly, but have different types of patients (women physicians have more female, minority and young patients). Women patients disclose more to women physicians, particularly for mental health, personal or sexually-related concerns. Women physicians are sued less frequently.

The NAMCS data provides some information on differences between how men and women practice medicine. In the 1977 survey (NAMCS 80-1710), selected diagnostic services ordered or provided were compared by sex of the physician for patients presenting with general symptoms and symptoms referable to the nervous, respiratory, digestive, genitourinary or musculoskeletal systems. "The only statistically significant result showed that female physicians were more likely to check blood pressure during visits for symptoms referring to the genitourinary system than were men." Thus, there appeared to be little difference between male and female physicians when dealing with the same type of patient. When comparing male and female physicians without controlling for diagnosis, the differences found in principal diagnosis were felt to reflect the different types of patient seen. There was little difference in the number of drugs prescribed except that male psychiatrists prescribed drugs more frequently than female psychiatrists. Women used blood pressure checks and PAP tests more frequently, again probably reflective of different patient populations (see chapter on Practice Characteristics). Proportionately more new patients were seen by the women, but male physicians saw more patients on referral than women. When asked to judge the seriousness of the patient's condition, male physicians believed their patients to be more seriously ill.

The 1980-81 NAMCS survey looked at specialty-specific differences. "Female Ob-Gyn's were more likely than male Ob-Gyn's to have new patients and to use PAP tests, laboratory tests, blood pressure checks, and diet counseling during visits." (NAMCS 84-1737) The female general and family practitioners ordered more PAP tests and clinical laboratory tests and provided more medical counseling (NAMCS 83-1734). Female pediatricians used general history and/or examination more frequently and had a higher proportion of visits that included blood pressure checks, diet counseling and family or social counseling (84-1737). They utilized drugs more frequently, although this had not been found to be true in the 1977 survey (NAMCS 80-1710) or for the obstetrician/gynecologists (NAMCS 84-1737) or general and family practitioners (NAMCS 83-1734). These specialty differences, however, were not controlled for differences in the patient populations of the male or females, and may result from the relatively higher proportions of new, women and/or younger patients in their practices. Similarly, Hartzema (1983) found physician sex did not explain differences in drug prescribing behavior when other factors were taken into account, and believed that physician sex in some earlier studies appeared to be important because physician sex was a proxy for differences in patient characteristics which had not be adequately taken into account.

Another study compared medical work-ups by 10 male and 10 female physicians for 142 male and 165 female patient visits in a health maintenance organization with chief complaints of chest pain, headache, dizziness, fatigue and back pain and found no difference in the extent of work-up nor the appropriateness of the work-up by sex of the physician or patient (Greer 1986).

Women physicians spend more time with their patients. The 1977 NAMCS survey (NAMCS 80-1710) reported that "the mean duration of all visits to women specialists was 17.8 minutes, compared with 15.3 to male specialists, which was chiefly due to the average time used by general and family practitioners (17.6 minutes for females in this specialty, compared to 12.7 minutes for males in the practice)." Similar longer duration visits were found in 1980-81 for general and family practitioners (NAMCS 83-1734), pediatricians (NAMCS 84-1736) and obstetrician/gynecologists (NAMCS 84-1737).

Women obstetrician/gynecologists are more likely to strongly believe that women should have the right to abortions, and are more likely to believe that Federal funds should pay for abortions (Weisman, FPP 1986). They are more likely to have gone into ob/gyn because of an interest in feminism or desire to improve health care for women (Margolis). Women obstetrician/gynecologists were also more likely to perform abortions, but averaged fewer abortions per provider than males (Weisman, FPP 1986). Women Ob/Gyn's were less likely to provide amniocentesis and artificial inseminations and some other infertility services (Weisman 1987).

A study by Schueneman (1985) found that women surgery residents (13 women representing 10% of the total in the study) were academically more qualified than men and did better on a visual perception task, but scored less well on a perceptual task involving both motor analysis and visual analysis in psychometric testing, which relates to operative skill, and were rated less well by their surgical superiors. The authors attributed this to potentially greater cautiousness in avoiding errors, and also noted that supervisors rated females less well in the area of confidence and task organization. The authors also quote another study (McGee) that found men to be more spatially and motorically proficient than women, although

McGee does not specify the amount of difference between the sexes. While this is a small number of women from which to generalize, and there was very little difference between the men and women (although a couple of the differences were statistically significant), this could suggest a complex mixture of effects creating a lack of confidence in surgical skills including greater cautiousness on the part of women in performing motor skills, contributing to less confidence in the training setting reinforced by generally male superiors.

Patients may be more likely to disclose mental illness symptoms or personal concerns to same-sex physicians (Young 1979). In reviewing the literature on disclosure of symptoms to physicians, Young (1979) noted that there was inconsistency in results, but believed that the major reason for this was that the studies had not taken into account what type of symptoms were to be disclosed.   When the type of symptom was determined, as in Young's study, greater disclosure to same-sex physician became more apparent.   An alternative explanation for inconsistency in this literature is the year the study was done and the experience rate of patients with male and female physicians. As fewer patients in earlier studies would have had the opportunity to see women physicians, their reaction may have been less positive (see Englemen). The concept of greater disclosure to same-sex physicians is reinforced by literature that has found that people will divulge more feelings to same-sex individuals in situations other than doctor-patient relationships (Highlen).

In another study (Riessman), women were more likely to disclose to male interviewers presumed to be lower status, and men to those of higher status. Similarly, Levinson (1984) found that men more strongly desired men physicians than women wanted women physicians, though both tended to want same-sex physicians, and that emotional problems or medical problems that required greater physical intimacy (complete physical exam, gynecological or prostate problem) also produced higher desires for same-sex physicians.

For genetic counseling, a female provider (not specifically physician) was better for female patients. When there was a female provider, there were more in-depth discussion, clearer explanations, and female patients were more likely to disclose concerns although the counseling sessions were similar in length (Zare 1984).

In a survey study of women physicians, Dickinson (1979) found that women physicians tended to relate better to dying patients and their families and become more depressed when the patient died.

Women physicians are sued less frequently (Medica, Sloan), probably because they perform fewer risky procedures (Ellsbury, Ogle) and possibly because of better doctor-patient relationships.

Broverman (1970) found that men and women physicians similarly stereotyped male and female patients. In rape counseling, women and men therapists essentially report similar treatment for victims; however, women rated the victims as more impaired, suggesting that they may have been more empathic with the victims (Bassuk).

Summary: Women as Healers

In general, male and female physicians appear to offer the same quality of care, performing similar medical work-ups for similar types of patients, while women physicians spend longer time with each patient and have more same-sex patients. Thus, the differences in care by women physicians and the impact of the differences are likely to be subtle, i.e., the within group variability is likely to be greater than the between group variability.

Weisman (1985) argues that physician gender may affect the quality of care through influences on 1) key characteristics of the doctor-patient relationship such as communication of information, the affective tone of the relationship and the negotiative quality of the relationship; 2) the expectations brought to the relationship by patients; and 3) the match in status of physician and patient in the relationship. Data suggests that there is greater disclosure in same-sex doctor-patient relationships, which generally would mean better care.

Women physicians are generally more oriented to the relationship, i.e., more 'nurturing.' Our own surmise is this is the reason that women physicians spend longer with their patients; they listen more to the personal issues and concerns of their patients and may spend more time counseling (an aspect of care which often does not end up recorded in charts). This may be the reason certain patients prefer women physicians.

The greater interest of the women physician in the relationship and the greater rapport between same-sex dyads would be most likely to help when patients state a preference for physician sex; when sexual, mental health or personal symptoms are treated; or when significant doctor-patient negotiation is required (see Weisman). However, in individual circumstances, the potential improvement could easily be overwhelmed by other important factors such as access or skill. Women physicians are generally less confident, or perhaps, said a different way, feel less 'strong' and 'active,' or less motivated to achieve. There is little research to suggest the impact of this on quality of care. It could mean more attention is taken in thinking through patient problems, which should improve outcome. Less risk taking lowers malpractice risk and decreases the risk to the patient, but could mean less gain for patients for whom the risk would have paid off. It may mean that the patient, in detecting the lower confidence, feels less secure, thus less readily cured through the placebo qualities of the doctor-patient relationship. It certainly means that women are less likely to strive for organizational and administrative leadership roles.

Many of the differences between men and women are socially reinforced. It would seem that potentiating the differences between the sexes by differential reward systems serves the functioning of society in some manner. Reinforcing differences between male and female physicians can also be positive, offering different opportunities for patients to maximize their own wishes in choice of physician.

On the whole, women and women physicians as compared to men and men physicians are 1) more oriented to relationships, with men more oriented to procedures; 2) more feminine or androgynous; 3) less confident in their abilities with equivalent training and intelligence; and 4) less motivated to achieve by traditional measures. Overall, women physicians are more different among themselves than between themselves and men physicians. Said another way, women physicians are similar to men physicians, but retain many characteristics attributed to women in our society (see also Weisman). Both men and women physicians represent subgroups of their sexes with some generalizable characteristics and much internal variability. Women offer much to medicine and may be the physicians of choice for many patients and situations.

References

Ackerman-Ross FS, Sochat N. Close encounters of the medical kind: Attitudes toward male and female physicians. Soc Sci Med 1980;14A:61-64. Bassuk E, Apsler R. Are there sex biases in rape counseling? Am J Psychiatry 1983;140(3):305-308.

Belenky MF, Clinchy BMcV, Goldberger NR, Tarule JM. Women's ways of knowing. Basic Books, Inc., New York, 1986.

Berquist SR, Duchac BW, Schalin VA et al. Perceptions of freshman medical students of gender differences in medical specialty choice. J Med Educ 1985;60:379-383.

Best DL, Williams JE, Briggs SR. A further analysis of the affective meanings associated with male and female sex-trait stereotypes. Sex Roles 1980;6(5): 735-746.

Broverman IK, Broverman DM, Clarkson FE, Rosenkrantz PS, Vogel SR. Sex-role stereotypes and clinical judgments of mental health. Journal of Consulting and Clinical Psychology 1970;34(1):1-7.

Broverman IK, Vogel SR, Broverman DM, Clarkson FE, Rosenkrantz PS. Sex-role stereotypes: A current appraisal. Journal of Social Issues 1972;28(2):59-78.

Campbell MA. Why would a girl go into medicine? The Feminist Press, New York, 1973.

Cartwright LK. Personality differences in male and female medical students. Psychiatry Med 1972;3:213-218.

Cartwright LK. Personality changes in a sample of women physicians. J Med Educ 1977;52:467-474.

Challacombe CB. Do women patients need women doctors? The Practitioner 1983; 227:848-850.

Clark DC, Zeldow PB. Vicissitudes of depressed mood during four years of medical school. JAMA 1988;260(17):2521-2528.

Coplin JW, Williams JE. Women law students' descriptions of self and the ideal lawyer. Psychology of Women Quarterly Summer 1978;2(4):323-333.

Crowson TW, Rich EC, Harris IB. A comparison of locus of control between men and women in an internal medicine residency. J Med Educ 1986;61:840-841.

Davis SW, Best DL, Marion G, Wall GH. Sex stereotypes in the self- and ideal descriptions of physician's assistant student. J Med Educ 1984;59:678-680.

Deaux K, Emswiller T. Explanations of successful performance on sex-linked tasks: What is skill for the male is luck for the female. Journal of Personality and Social Psychology 1974;29(1):80-85.

Deaux K, White L, Farris E. Skill versus luck: Field and laboratory studies of male and female preferences. Journal of Personality and Social Psychology 1975;32(4): 629-636.

Dickinson GE, Pearson AA. Sex differences of physicians in relating to dying patients. J Am Med Wom Assoc 1979;34:45-47.

Ellsbury K, Schneeweiss R, Montano DE, Gordon KC, Kuykendall D. Gender differences in practice characteristics of graduates of family medicine residencies. J Med Educ 1987;62:895-903.

Engleman EG. Attitudes toward women physicians. A study of 500 clinic patients. West J Med 1974;120:95-100.

Feather NT. Attribution of responsibility and valence of success and failure in relation to initial confidence and task performance. Journal of Personality and Social Psychology 1969;13(2):129-144.

Feather NT, Simon JG. Reactions to male and female success and failure in sex-linked occupations: Impressions of personality, causal attributions, and perceived likelihood of different consequences. Journal of Personality and Social Psychology 1975;31(1):20-31.

Feldman-Summers S, Kiesler SB. Those who are number two try harder: The effect of sex on attributions of causality. Journal of Personality and Social Psychology 1974;30(6):846-855.

Fenton WS, Robinowitz CB, Leaf PJ. Male and female psychiatrists and their patients. Am J Psychiatry 1987;144(3):358-361.

Fiorentine R. Men, women and the premed persistence gap: A normative alternatives approach. American Journal of Sociology 1987;92(5):1118-1139.

Frey J, Demick J, Bibace R. Variations in physicians' feeling of control during a family practice residency. J Med Educ 1981;56:50-56.

Frieze IH, Whitley BE, Hanusa BH, McHugh MC. Assessing the theoretical models for sex differences in causal attributions for success and failure. Sex Roles 1982;8(4):333-343.

Gilligan C. In a different voice. Harvard University Press, Cambridge, Massachusetts 1982.

Giles H, Williams JE. Medical students' descriptions of self and ideal physician. Soc Sci Med 1979;13A:813-815.

Greer S, Dickerson V, Schneiderman LJ, Atkins C, Bass R. Responses of male and female physicians to medical complaints in male and female patients. J Fam Pract 1986;23(1):49-53.

Gross W, Crovitz E. A comparison of medical students' attitudes toward women and women medical students. J Med Educ 1975;50:392-394.

Haar E, Halitsky V, Stricker G. Factors related to the preference for a female gynecologist. Med Care 1975;13(9):782-790.

Hartzema AG, Christensen DB. Nonmedical factors associated with the prescribing volume among family practitioners in an HMO. Med Care 1983;21(10):990-1000.

Highlen PS, Gillis SF. Effects of situational factors, sex, and attitude on affective self-disclosure and anxiety. Journal of Counseling Psychology 1978;25(4):270-276.

Hoffman DM, Fidell LS. Characteristics of androgynous, undifferentiated, masculine, and feminine middle-class women. Sex Roles 1979;5(6):765-781.

Hoffman LW. Early childhood experiences and women's achievement motives. Journal of Social Issues 1972;28(2):129-155.

Jacklin CN. Methodological issues in the study of sex-related differences. Developmental Review 1981;1:266-273.

Kasteler JM, Humle S. Attitudes toward women physicians in a Mormon community. J Am Med Wom Assoc 1980;35(2):37-41.

Lenney E. Women's self-confidence in achievement settings. Psychological Bulletin 1977;84(1):1-13.

Leserman J. Men and women in medical school: How they change and how they compare. Praeger, New York, 1981.

Levinson RM, McCollum KT, Kutner NG. Gender homophily in preferences for physicians. Sex Roles 1984;10(5/6):315-325.

Lorber J. Women physicians: Careers, status, and power. Tavistock Publications, New York, 1984.

Maheux B, Dufort F, Beland F. Professional and sociopolitical attitudes of medical students: Gender differences reconsidered. J Am Med Wom Assoc 1988;43(3):73-76.

McGee MG. Human spatial abilities: Psychometric studies and environmental, genetic, hormonal, and neurological influences. Psychological Bulletin 1979;86(5):889-918.

Medica. Women doctors sued less often. Winter 1983:29-30.

National Ambulatory Medical Care Survey, United States, 1977. Characteristics of visits to female and male physicians. U.S. Department of Health and Human Services, Public Health Service, Office of Health Research, Statistics, and Technology, National Center for Health Statistics. Publication No. (PHS) 80-1710, Hyattsville, MD, June 1980.

National Ambulatory Medical Care Survey, United States, January 1980-December 1981. Patterns of ambulatory care in general and family practice. U.S. Department of Health and Human Services, Public Health Service, National

Center for Health Statistics. Publication No. (PHS) 83-1734, Hyattsville, MD, September 1983.

National Ambulatory Medical Care Survey, United States, January 1980-December 1981. Patterns of ambulatory care in pediatrics. U.S. Department of Health and Human Services, Public Health Service, National Center for Health Statistics, publication No. (PHS) 84-1736, Hyattsville, MD, October 1983.

National Ambulatory Medical Care Survey, United States, January 1980-December 1981. Patterns of ambulatory care in obstetrics and gynecology. U.S. Department of Health and Human Services, Publication No. (PHS) 84-1737, Hyattsville, MD, February 1984.

Needle RH, Murray BA. The relationship between race and sex of health provider, the quality of care provided, and levels of satisfaction with gynecological care among black college women. Coll Health December 16, 1977;127-131.

Ogle KS, Henry RC, Durda K, Zivick JD. Gender-specific differences in family practice graduates. J Fam Pract 1986;23(4):357-360.

Petravage JB, Reynolds LJ, Gardner HJ, Reading JC. Attitudes of women toward the gynecologic examination. J Fam Pract 1979;9(6):1039-1045.

Philliber SG, Jones J. Staffing a contraceptive service for adolescents: The importance of sex, race, and age. Public Health Reports 1982;97(2):165-169.

Restak R. We need more cheap, docile women doctors. Washington Post, Sunday, April 27, 1986.

Rezler AG, Buckley JM. A comparison of personality types among female student health professionals. J Med Educ 1977;52:475-477.

Riessman CK. Interview effects in psychiatric epidemiology: A study of medical and lay interviewers and their impact on reported symptoms. Am J Public Health 1979;69(5):485-491.

Roessler R, Collins F, Mefferd RB, Jr. Sex similarities in successful medical school applicants. J Am Med Wom Assoc 1975;30(6):254-265.

Ross CE, Mirowsky J, Duff RS. Physician status characteristics and client satisfaction in two types of medical practice. Journal of Health and Social Behavior 1982;23:317-329.

Russo NF, Denmark FL. Women, psychology, and public policy. American Psychologist 1984;39(10):1161-1165.

Schueneman AL, Pickleman J, Freeark RJ. Age, gender, lateral dominance, and prediction of operative skill among general surgery residents. Surgery 1985;98(3):506-513.

Seymore C, DuRant RH, Jay MS, Freeman D, et al. Influence of position during examination, and sex of examiner on patient anxiety during pelvic examination. J Pediatr 1986;108:312-317.

Shapiro J, McGrath E, Anderson RC. Patients', medical students', and physicians' perceptions of male and female physicians. Perceptual and Motor Skills 1983;56:179-190.

Sloan FA, Mergenhagen PM, Burfield WB, Bovbjerg RR, Hassan M. Medical malpractice experience of physicians: Predictable or haphazard? JAMA 1989;262(23):3291-3297.

Weisman CS, Nathanson CA, Teitelbaum MA, Chase GA, King TM. Abortion attitudes and performance among male and female obstetrician-gynecologists. Family Planning Perspectives 1986;18(2):67-73.

Weisman CS, Nathanson CA, Teitelbaum MA, Chase GA, King TM. Delivery of fertility control services by male and female obstetrician-gynecologists. Am J Obstet Gynecol 1987;156:464-469.

Weisman CS, Teitelbaum MA. Physician gender and the physician-patient relationship: Recent evidence and relevant questions. Soc Sci Med 1985;20(11): 1119-1127.

Williams JE, Best DL. Sex stereotypes in education, occupation, and mental health. In Williams and Best, Measuring sex stereotypes: A thirty nation study. Sage Publications 1982:289-303.

Williams JE, Best DL. Measuring sex stereotypes. Revised Edition, Sage Publications 1990.

Willoughby L, Calkins V, Arnold L. Different predictors of examination performance for male and female medical students. J Am Med Wom Assoc 1979;34(8): 316-320.

Young JW. Symptom disclosure to male and female physicians: Effects of sex, physical attractiveness, and symptom type. Journal of Behavioral Medicine 1979;2(2):159-169.

Zare N, Sorenson JR, Heeren T. Sex of provider as a variable in effective genetic counseling. Soc Sci Med 1984;19(7):671-675.

"Women physicians are different in many important characteristics from their male counterparts. As the proportion of women in all types of roles of the physician universe increases, the image of physicians, the nature of their work, and the structure of their organizations will change.

The basis for my observation is a 20-year opportunity to work with a substantial number of women physicians in a variety of health policy administrative roles. Although most analyses of the impact of increasing numbers of women physicians have focused on productivity, I believe the most significant differences lie not in how much women physicians do, but how they approach their tasks.

There is a growing body of literature suggesting that personality types and interpersonal styles of women physicians differ from that of their male colleagues. My anecdotal observations would be consistent with this, and I would note that, in particular, women physicians in leadership roles seem to be far more likely to adopt strategies of consensus building rather than competition. Since an increasing number of studies in the field of organizational development and behavior suggest that the most successful organizations will be those in which "win-win" solutions are established to resolve competing interests, the different approaches to leadership by women physicians suggests that their impact as individuals and institutions in which they serve may far outweigh their absolute numbers."

Dr. Robert Graham

(Dr. Graham is a physician who has been primarily involved in health policy administration. After serving 12 years with the United States Public Health Service, he now is the Executive Vice President of the American Academy of Family Physicians. He has been married for 14 years to another physician-administrator-clinician, Dr. Jane Henney).

8
Physician Stress

When a hungry saber-toothed tiger came upon a cavewoman, eying her as his next meal, the cavewomen experienced the "fight or flight" response: her heart pounded in her chest, she began to breathe rapidly and her muscles tensed in preparation for her planned escape. The stronger such response, the more likely she was to escape from the danger; thus, this response appears to have given her a distinct evolutionary advantage. Even today, this response is common and integral to our lives. Though there are no longer saber-toothed tigers, the prehistoric stress response remains, a much cited factor in both medical and lay literature. Estimates are that, due to stress, between 50 and 75 billion dollars a year are lost on absenteeism, medical expenses and decreased productivity in the United States (Wallis).

To understand stress as is meant today, a better definition than "fight or flight" is needed. Dr. Hans Selye (1976), the 'father of stress,' has defined it as the nonspecific response of the body to any change or demand. This means any change, positive or negative, in a person's life can induce stress. Even the seemingly minor hassles of daily living can add up to a substantial stress response. In fact, the stress of daily living may have a more damaging effect on a person's well-being than a major life change. Overall, however, all stress is in some sense additive, since it occurs in an individual who is continuously adapting to past and existing stress.

Research on Stress

There has been much research (Selye) on the chemistry of stress in the past several years. Examination of brain tissue after physical stress has revealed that levels of norepinephrine dropped 20% and of epinephrine between 30 and 40%. Stress also boosted the production of endorphins which may be the body's natural method for raising its threshold of pain. This alteration of the body's chemistry by stress may well initiate or potentiate the development of many diseases, including psychiatric disorders. For example, depression has been associated with low levels of norepinephrine and serotonin. It is also known that the body's immune response, including T-lymphocytes, are inhibited by chronic stress.

Our stressful life-style is a principle cause of illness. Somewhere between one-half and two-thirds of office visits to primary care physicians are prompted by stress-related illnesses. Stress is thought to contribute to coronary artery disease, peptic ulcer disease, asthma, and injuries on the job, and may indirectly contribute to cirrhosis of the liver and such diverse conditions as herpes, multiple sclerosis and many other illnesses (Wallis). It is surely a sign of our times that some of the best-selling drugs in our country today are ulcer drugs and minor tranquilizers.

The stressful combination of high demands and low conn
trol over one's job raise the risk of heart disease as much as smoking or high cholesterol. Karasek, from Columbia University, found that workers such as cooks and garment stitchers who worked on an assembly line and had little control over their jobs, but high demands, developed heart disease at a very high rate (Wallis). This has been corroborated in a cross-sectional design study of Swedish workers with high demand, low control and low social support, revealing about twice the prevalence of cardiovascular disease as in workers with low demand, high control and high social support, after controlling for 11 other potential factors (Johnson).

Dr. Neal Miller of Rockefeller University did a classic study on control and stress (Wallis). He subjected a group of rats to a series of electrical shocks. The first group was provided with a way to control the timing of the shocks; the second group was unable to control the timing. Both groups received the same total number of shocks, but the group with no control developed five times the number of stomach ulcerations as those with control. This is consistent with the concept that control of a stressful situation reduces its negative effects.

Dorian and Garfinkel (1987) reviewed the literature on stress and illness. They believe that the most convincing literature relates stress to infectious illnesses, such as colds, in humans and in animal experimental models, but that there is sufficient evidence to believe there is also a relationship between stress, altered immunity and illness. They note that acute stress is probably different than chronic stress. However, the relationships are probably complex, rather than simple, and the literature contains contradictory information, probably as a result of differing definitions of stress, lack of control groups, and other methodological problems. As a example of variant information, a recent 10-year follow-up of Finnish workers found no relationship between initial stress symptoms and mortality (Aro).

One of the ways to consider the stress/illness connection is to look at stress-related psychiatric illnesses. Depression is one psychiatric illness that is linked to stress (Gold), and appears to be more clearly linked to other medical illnesses than other types of psychiatric illnesses (Dorian and Garfinkel). Recent data (Bruce) found that the odds of dying were four times greater for those with affective illnesses, controlling for age, sex, and physical health. However, this does not appear to be due to cancer, according to the study (Zonderman).

One psychological factor that has received a lot of attention is the Type A personality (Friedman). First identified by San Francisco cardiologists, Drs. Friedman and Rosenman, Type A behavior is characterized by the tendency to try to accomplish too many things in too little time. Secondarily, Type As appear to exhibit a great deal of hostility. Most Type A people get irritated at trivial things; they are very competitive at work and at home. Type A personalities tend to produce 40 times as much cortisol and four times as much epinephrine as the Type B personalities, who are less competitive, more contemplative, and less oriented to time (Selye).

Stress Curve

The stress curve is a useful model for understanding stress and its effects (see Fig 8-1). The X axis on the graph represents the amount of stress or change a person is experiencing. Note that there is no point on the graph where stress is nonexistent. The Y axis represents productivity. To a certain point on the graph, the old adage that "stress is good for you" applies. As stress increases, productivity also rises. After a certain critical point, however, increased stress does not increase productivity. If stress continues to increase, fatigue intervenes and productivity decreases. After a person moves into the fatigue area, further stress causes exhaustion which can lead to ill-health or burnout. In exhaustion, there is no reserve for dealing with added stress (Nixon).

The amount of stress an individual can tolerate is influenced by many factors including their nutritional state, their level of fatigue, and the adequacy of their coping skills (Murphy). (See Fig. 8-2.) While the stress curve is probably simplistic (King), it does help us to think about the potential, but varying, impacts of stressful events on our lives.

Stress and the Medical Student

Though stress in the 1990s is a universal disease, there are aspects of medicine that are uniquely stressful. The process begins with medical training. All medical students must make a transition from their previous lives to the realities of being a medical student. As such, all face stressors that have the potential for being disruptive to their lives, or for providing motivation for greater achievement and self-fulfillment. Medical students

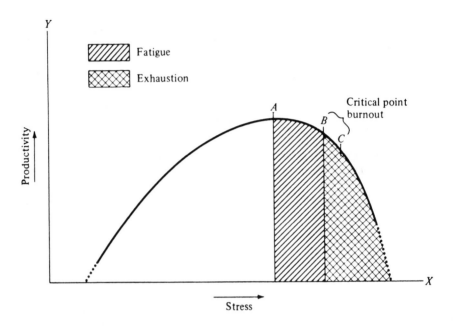

FIGURE 8-1 The Stress Curve. (Adapted with permission from Practitioner, Vol 935, The Human Function Curve: With Special Reference to: Cardiovascular Disorders, 1976.)

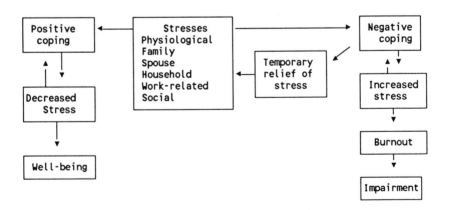

FIGURE 8-2 Stress Cycle

perceive medical school to be significantly different than undergraduate school (Gottheil), often in desirable ways.

In one study (Coburn), first-year medical students gave the following factors the eight highest mean stress scores:

1.   Final examinations;
2.   Fear of the inability to absorb the amount of course material;
3.   Fear of bad grades;
4.   The huge number of hours needed to study;
5.   The limited recreational and social outlets;
6.   Lack of sexual outlets;
7.   The feeling of loneliness; and
8.   Initial dissection experience with a cadaver.

The following were the six most frequently ranked sources of stress anticipated for later in their careers:

1.   Death of a patient;
2.   Fear of error in diagnosis and treatment;
3.   Dealing with a patient with a chronic or helpless disease;
4.   Fear for personal health in contact with sick people;
5.   Discussion with patients about marital or sexual problems; and
6.   Carrying out physical exams.

Obviously, the medical students were concerned with the possible inability to grasp and absorb all the materials that were being presented to them. But the stresses were not academic alone. It is obvious that the students' lack of social contact also served as a source of stress. They experienced feelings of inadequacy and incompetence. The authors believed that damage was done to the self-image of the medical students, producing serious stress reactions and possibly serious consequences for the student's continued education. 40% of one medical school class (Boyle) admitted considering quitting.

In another study (Woods), medical students feared they had developed the diseases they learned about in medical school, resulting in hypochondriasis or "medical students' disease," and that many students found their fears significantly stressful.

However, one should not conclude that medical school is uniquely more stressful than other graduate schools; law students and graduate psychology students report higher stress scores than medical students (Heins 1984).

This was despite of the substantially higher number of hours that medical students spent working on academics.

Stress for Women in Medical School

First year medical students in Toronto (Coburn) felt that the academic factors were the most stressful and social factors the least stressful; women found the academics more stressful than the men did.   Many women graduate students, including medical students, face "crises in their personal lives as well as severe reality problems dealing with dual roles, finances, uncertain job market, child care problems, etc." (Kaplan)   Spiegel (1987) found that women medical students were more stressed than men by conflicts with authorities, and responded by applying more effort to school. At the University of Texas, women had more depression and anxiety during the first year (Lloyd).   Women were more stressed by lack of time, deadline and difficulties in personal relationships in another study (Clark). These same women more often said that their personal relationships had ended.   Women are the minority in medical schools, and the stresses of being a minority are probably operative (Bowers, Hilberman).   In particular, feelings of isolation (Hoferek) and loneliness are common for minority groups. However, the association between grades and stress was a positive one for women (Spiegel 1986).

Discrimination exists in medical schools against women medical students.   In fact, an entire book has been written on the discrimination perceived by women (Campbell). The amount of discrimination perceived is variable by the individual woman's antenna.   One study of attitudes toward women physicians in medical academia (Scadron) found that male medical students were the least supportive of women physicians as leaders or of increasing the number of women in the class to half.   In another study (Grant), however, women students reported that the male faculty members exhibited the most sexism.

Stress is ubiquitous and can have negative consequences (see also chapter 6 on Mental Health).   Several small studies have looked at the utilization of health services or counseling by men and women medical students, each concluding that women seek services more frequently then men.   Heins (1979) noted that women at the medical school had more health and identity/personal problems than did the men; however, the office that reported the work and handled the problems was entirely staffed by women, which may have inhibited men from using the services. The author also concluded that the women had a greater ability to deal with their problems than men. Davidson (1978) reported that 21% of the women students and 6% of the male students utilized the student psychiatric health service which was staffed by one male and one female psychiatrist, with the most common problems being adjustment and situational reactions, marital dysfunction and neurotic and character problems. The students in their basic science years made more use of the service than those in the clinical years, similar to the findings of Adsett (1968), that first year students were the heaviest users of health services. Adsett (1968) also found that women used the counseling services more than men, but attributed this to their greater ability to ask for help, as also reported by another study (Cleary).

Stress and the Resident

The issue of resident stress has jumped to the forefront of critical issues facing medicine in the last several years. The controversy surrounding the Libby Zion case in New York (McCall 1988) sparked an avalanche of literature on resident stress in both the medical and lay literature. The resulting public fears about the quality of care given by overworked residents has resulted in legislation regulating resident work hours in New York and attempts by many other states to enact similar laws (Colford). The multiple stresses of residency training are being examined carefully and may result in strategies to help improve our current medical education system.

Issues facing residents are similar to those of other young professionals. Residents and other young human services professionals share almost identical responses to stresses, including issues of personal development, changes in their lives, constant patient responsibility and burnout (Cherniss). Residents may be particularly vulnerable to depression (see Chapter 6 on Mental Health).

Resident stresses are also similar to those of physicians (Mawardi), although the experience of the stress may be different. For example, both residents and practicing physicians find difficult patients stressful. However, the resident has the added stress of not being the patient's primary doctor and not knowing the patient before the medical encounter.

Issues particularly difficult for the residency years include sleep deprivation, lack of personal time, indebtedness, and the educational system itself.

Sleep Deprivation Sleep deprivation is believed to be the greatest source of stress during a residency. The resident on call averages 122-273 minutes of sleep (Lurie). Studies of the effects of sleep deprivation, however, are contradictory and incomplete. Friedman (1973) found an increased rate of electrocardiogram reading errors with sleep deprivation. No decrease in mathematical skills were found in another study (Leighton). A 1988 study of surgery residents (Deaconson) claimed no difference in the sleep deprived state for resident performance on psychometric testing. However, the residents were on call every other night, and the control residents were those who had not been on call the night before, but still probably sleep deprived. Storer (1989) found no effect of sleep deprivation on the cognitive skill of pediatric residents but a decreased ability to perform coordinated tasks. Thus, the effects of sleep deprivation on actual patient care is unknown, and further testing outside the artificial cognitive test environment is needed (Wagner).

Lack of Personal Time Residents, because of long work hours, have little time for family, friendships, hobbies and personal activities (Ford, Hinz). A direct result of this can be feelings of isolation, loneliness or inadequacy (Freidman 1973).

Indebtedness The rising debt resulting from increased medical education costs is a source of stress to residents. The average debt of a graduating medical student is over $32,000 (estimated by the Association of American Medical Colleges) and may reach as high as $50,000 shortly after 1990 (Blackwell, Sandson). To ease the debt, 33-80% of residents moonlight (McCue), potentially compounding the problem of sleep deprivation.

Educational System The medical education system as been described as "a neglectful and abusive family system" (McKegney) with unrealistic expectations, denial, indirect communication patterns, rigidity and isolation. Continuing this parallel, like parents who raise their children as they themselves were raised, each generation of educators teach as they were taught (McKegney).

There are many examples of the types of problems that occur. Residents are rudely awakened when on call. Time spent on formal teaching is often sporadic and unstructured (Cook). There is frequently little time for indepth reading. Residents are frequently faced with ethical dilemmas with little or no training in ethical issues. "Pimping" the resident remains a traditional way of teaching. Pimping is the method of asking difficult questions to lower level residents with the intent of embarrassing them, often leading to low self-esteem (Brancati). "Scut" work--nonmedical patient-related tasks--increases the workload of residents. With increased cost-cutting measures on the part of hospitals, the amount of scut work, such as patient transportation, for residents may be increasing (Glickman, Smith). Intensive care and emergency room rotations may be more stressful (Schwartz).

Resident Marriages Marital distress among residents has not been well studied. In his book on physician marriages, Myers (1988) noted a fifth of married residents cite communication difficulties, lack of time with spouse, arguments over finances, work and sharing of domestic responsibilities, and concerns about sexual relationships. Similarly Landau found 40% of residents to have significant marital problems; three-quarters of the residents blamed the problems on the residency.

Women Residents Women residents feel more stress in their personal lives and more frequently seek counseling than men residents (Janus). Women residents also feel more stress in the multiple roles they must assume (Coombs). Young (1987) found a higher incidence of maladaptive coping behaviors (including alcohol use) and emotional problems in women than men residents.

In a recent survey of 1,120 women residents by Dickstein (Page), almost a quarter complained of sexual come-ons by patients, one in five of sexual harassment by their attending physicians, and a tenth of having no friends. To compound the feelings of loneliness, the significant others of half of the unmarried women lived in another city.

Potential Solutions Various solutions to the stresses of residency has been suggested. Work hours (McCall 1989) and scut work could be reduced. Residents could be more directly supervised on all shifts (McCall 1989). Moonlighting could be restricted, or perhaps discouraged by increasing salaries (McCall 1989). Formal mechanisms for early detection and intervention should be in place (McCue). Formal support groups for residents or their spouses are helpful (McCue, Colford, Reuben 1984). Other innovative ways of dealing with current problems, such as night-float systems or backup systems in case of resident illness, have also been suggested (Schwartz).

Stress and the Physician

After the doctor finishes full-time medical education and enters practice, there are new stressors, often revolving around intensely emotional issues that are governed by strong cultural codes (McCue 1982). The physician is forced to deal with such issues as difficult patients, sexuality, death, hostile families, difficult diagnostic problems, unrealistic expectations, and the changing milieu of medicine, often without adequate training (McCue 1982, Spears). Each of these will be discussed in more depth.

Difficult Patients When students enter medicine, they expect that they will be helping people and be satisfied by the relationships that they develop with their patients. They are often sorely disappointed when they routinely start seeing patients who are anxious, uncomfortable and/or hostile. Instead of the multitude of unusual and exciting illnesses that are pounded into the medical student's head in school, the ultimate reason for a large number of patients seeking care is a fear of an illness, rather than the rare disease itself. The 'worried well' are often fatiguing and unpleasant (Spears). These difficult patients are a source of stress.

Sexuality The stress of dealing with human sexuality and the resultant embarrassment is always present, no matter how experienced the clinician is. There is always the desire to preserve modesty accompanied by the need to acquire clinical information (Spears). Medical students are at greatest risk for the stress of embarrassment concerning sexuality because they must delve into these areas without the full privilege of the physician (McCue 1982). Yet, each student and physician must forge ahead in spite of embarrassment because missing data could result in an even worse stress--guilt (McCue 1982).

Death Though death is the natural outcome of many of the illnesses physician treat, death is still seen by the medical profession as a failure. It is an emotional issue in any event. Physicians also area responsible for making life-and-death decisions, including the connection or disconnection of life-supporting machines (McCue 1982, Spears), godlike decisions frequently made without firm societal backing.

Hostile Families Death or ongoing illness can be seen by the patient's family as a failure of the physician. It is not uncommon for a family member to turn on the physician with verbal or legal hostility, for whatever the reason, when the patient outcome was not ideal.

Difficult Diagnostic Problems Most people enter medicine with the pre-conceived notion that medicine is an exacting science where everything is black or white. By the end of training, they realize it is actually a world of gray: it is necessary to make clinical decisions on the basis of conflicting or incomplete data, as well as considering the cost of the various treatments.

Unrealistic Expectations Not only do physicians usually enter medicine presuming they will cure, but the patients also share the same belief. The public is bombarded daily by the media with information about miracle cures and new technology that will save them. Thus, they expect to be healed, when generally, cures are not possible. The physician frequently cannot live up to the expectations placed on her/him, and stress results.

Malpractice The increased incidence of malpractice suits and the large dollar awards are affecting the daily working decisions and lives of physicians. Some are changing their specialties or work habits because of high malpractice insurance premiums. The Federal government is starting a nationwide computer information service to keep track of all actions (malpractice and adverse hospital privilege actions) taken against physicians.

Of physicians who are sued, only 4% state they had no physical or emotional reaction to being sued (Charles 1984); 39% had symptoms suggestive of a major depressive disorder; 20% had cluster or anger symptoms; 15% had the onset or exacerbation of physical illness during the period of litigation; a few percent had suicidal ideation or alcohol or drug misuse. In a Chicago Medical Society survey, a quarter of the physicians who had been sued noted that this was the single most stressful period in their lives (Charles 1987).

Changing Medical Milieu Changes are stressful, and the world of medicine is changing rapidly. Medicine is becoming more businesslike, industrialized, and decisions are frequently made on an economic basis. The result is that physicians will have less control over their work lives. Additionally, there are more and more constraints on how medicine is practiced: insurance companies provide criteria by which physicians must practice; peer review organizations often appear to have arbitrary criteria. The world of medicine in the next century will surely be a new one.

Reactions to Physician Stress

Doctors, along with society, aspire to deny the effects of stress. After having spent 30 years of their lives becoming physicians, they tend to be reluctant to acknowledge the discomfort caused them by their profession (McCue 1982, Tokarz). Instead of using positive coping mechanisms as described in the chapter on Stress Prevention and Management, physicians may employ negative coping mechanisms.

Negative coping is, by definition, detrimental. If an individual uses negative coping skills she/he steps on a merry-go-round. While negative coping may reduce stress on an immediate, but temporary, basis, unfortunately, it does not address the underlying stress that is the cause of the behavior, actually perpetuating and intensifying the stress. Examples of negative coping mechanisms are substance abuse, risk taking, and psychosomatic illness. Someone using drugs, such as marijuana or cocaine, may feel good at the time, or may enjoy the company of fellow drug users, but the underlying stressful responses to overwork or insecurity in dealing with patients or other factors continues unabated.

There appears to be a particular set of negative coping mechanisms used by physicians. Although many are probably already in use by the time the physician begins medical school, the current system of medical training may unfortunately reinforce their use. The most common negative coping behaviors used by physicians are:

Isolation from Family A common reaction to stress in the physician is to retreat from family life in order to meet the demands of medical practice (Fine). There is, in fact, an emotional separation from family life in the early years of practice, with home activities frequently interrupted by telephones and pagers. This erodes the time and energy needed for the interpersonal relationships of the physician (McCue 1984, Tokarz). However, the 'self-sacrificing' physician who surrenders her/his personal life and family life to the patient may well earn respect from colleagues (Spears). Doctors also receive a lot of positive strokes in their work environment. It is ego-gratifying to issue orders, make critical decisions, receive praise from patients and personnel and be treated as an important person. This compounds the problem of returning home, where the physician is just another wife or husband (McCue 1984, Tokarz).

Social Isolation Social isolation is another reaction to stress. It may well be a response to 'role fatigue' (Haleran). The physician may cease to interact socially with others, feeling that it takes time and effort she/he does not have, thus shutting themselves off from the support that others can provide. They may also permit themselves to be 'on-duty' at parties--answering medical questions, not relaxing, always being 'the physician'.

Burnout Burnout has had multiple definitions (Wessells), but could be called "absence of vision" or "when you are no longer effective and you no longer care" (Selder), a professional ennui (Regelson). Burnout is related to impairment, but generally refers to an emotional reaction to continually giving and providing care to others to the extent that the physician loses empathy and interest in helping patients or clients.

Impairment Another reaction to stress is impairment. Some estimates are that 10% of the physician population is 'impaired' (Coping). A physician is considered impaired when a personal problem interferes with the quality of medical care, the physician's education, family life or the physician's well-being. These dramatic outcomes seem to be the end stage of a process which at first has much milder symptoms and signs. Unfortunately, however, patterns often develop and proliferate many years before friends, colleagues or the public are aware of the doctor's problem or the probable consequences (Coping).

Other negative coping mechanisms used by physicians include:

1. Alcohol or drug abuse.
2. Promiscuity. If the basic needs for social interaction, sexuality, and self-esteem are not adequately met, promiscuity is a way of developing 'fleeting intimacy.'
3. Anger at patients. When stress becomes overwhelming, the physician may misdirect her/his anger at the patient, who becomes the enemy.
4. Preoccupation with illness/decreased empathy. Being preoccupied with 'the gallbladder in room 124' allows the physician to avoid the stress of dealing with the patient as a human being.
5. Sarcasm/cynicism. Sarcasm is thinly veiled hostility. What appears to be a cynical joke may be poor coping as opposed to a witty personality.

More on the mental health of physicians is summarized in Chapter 6.

Summary

Stress is ubiquitous and can help an individual move forward in her/his life, motivating a person to do wonderful things, or lead to illness, fatigue, burnout, or impairment. Physicians have some unique stresses related to their profession and can utilize positive or negative coping mechanisms to deal with them.

References

Adsett CA. Psychological health of medical students in relation to the medical education process. J Med Educ 1968;43:728-734.

Aro S, Hasan J. Occupational class, psychosocial stress and morbidity. Annals of Clinical Research 1987;19(2):62-68.

Blackwell B. Prevention of impairment among residents in training. JAMA 1986; 255:1177-1178.

Bowers JZ. Special problems of women medical students. J Med Educ 1968; 43:532-537.

Boyle BP, Coombs RH. Personality profiles related to emotional stress in the initial year of medical training. J Med Educ 1971;56:882-888.

Brancati FL. The art of pimping. JAMA 1989;262:89-90.

Bruce ML, Leaf PJ. Psychiatric disorders and 15-month mortality in a community sample of older adults. Am J Public Health 1989;79:727-730.

Campbell MA. Why would a girl go into medicine? New York, The Feminist Press 1973.

Charles SC, Warnecke RB, Wilbert JR, Lichtenberg R, DeJesus C. Sued and nonsued physicians: Satisfactions, dissatisfactions, and sources of stress. Psychosomatics 1987;28(9):462-466.

Charles SC, Wilbert JR, Kennedy EC. Physician's self reports of reactions to malpractice litigation. Am J Psychiatry 1984;141:563-565.

Cherniss C. Professional burnout in human service organizations. Praeger Publishers, New York, 1980, p. 41.

Clark EJ, Ricker PP. Gender differences in relationships and stress of medical and law students. J Med Educ 1986;61:32-40.

Cleary PD. Gender differences in stress-related disorders. In Gender & Stress, Barnett RC, Biener L, Baruch GK, eds., The Free Press, Macmillan, Inc., New York, 1987.

Coburn D, Jovaisas AV. Perceived sources of stress among first year medical students. J Med Educ 1975;50:589-595.

Colford JM, McPhee SJ. Ravelled sleeve of care. JAMA 1989;261:889-893.

Cook M. Stress and coping in internal medicine residency. West J Med 1986;142: 547-548.

Coombs RH, Hovanessian HC. Stress in the role constellation of female resident physicians. J Am Med Wom Assoc 1988;43:21-27.

Coping, Stress and the Practicing Physician--A workshop, 1981. Scientific Assembly, American Academy of Family Physicians.

Davidson V. Coping styles of women medical students. J Med Educ 1978;53: 902-907.

Deaconson TF, O'Hait DP, Levy MF, et al. Sleep deprivation and resident performance. JAMA 1988;260:1721-1727.

Dorian B, Garfinkel PE. Stress, immunity and illness--A review. Psychological Medicine 1987;17:393-407.

Fine C. Married to medicine: An intimate portrait of doctors' wives. Athenium, NY, 1981.

Ford CV, Wentz DK. Internship: What is stressful? S Med J 1986;79:595-599.

Freidman RC, Kornfeld DS, Bigger TJ. Psychological problems associated with sleep deprivation in interns. J Med Educ 1973;48:436-441.

Freidman RC, Bigger TJ, Kornfeld DS. The intern and sleep loss. N Engl J Med 1971;285:201-203.

Friedman M, Roseman R. Type A behavior and your heart. Alfred A. Knopf, NY, 1974, p 276.

Glickman R. Housestaff training: The need for careful reform. N Engl J Med 1988;318:780-782.

Gottheil E, Thornton CC, Conly SS, Cornelison FS, Jr. Stress, satisfaction, and performance: Transition from university to medical college. J Med Educ 1969; 44:270-277.

Grant L. The gender climate of medical school. J Am Med Wom Assoc 1988;43: 109-119.

Haleran JF. Doctors don't have to burn out. Medical Economics Oct 26, 1981: 148-161.

Heins M, Fahey SN, Leiden LI. Perceived stress in medical, law, and graduate students. J Med Educ 1984;59:169-179.

Heins M, Thomas J. Women medical students: A new appraisal. J Am Med Wom Assoc 1979;34(11):408-415.

Hilberman E, Konan J, Perez-Reyes M, et al. Support groups for women in medical school: A first-year program. J Med Educ 1975;50:867-875.

Hinz CA. Stress among resident on rise. Am Med News, July 22/29, 1983, p. 1-8.

Hoferek MJ, Sarnowski AA. Feelings of loneliness in women medical students. J Med Educ 1981;56:397-403.

Janus L, et al. Residents: The pressure's on the women. J Am Med Wom Assoc 1983;38:18-21.

Johnson JV, Hall EM. Job strain, workplace social support, and cardiovascular disease: A cross-sectional study of a random sample of the Swedish working population. Am J Public Health 1988;78:1336-1342.

Kaplan LH, Pao M. Problems facing women students in schools of medicine, law and business. JACH 1977;36:76-78.

King M, Stanley G, Burrows G. Stress: Theory and practice. Grune & Stratton, Inc., Orlando, FL, 1987.

Landau C, Hall S, et al. Stress in social and family relationships during medical residency. J Med Educ 1986;61:654-660.

Leighton K, Livingston M. Fatigue in doctors. Lancet 1983;1:1280.

Lloyd C, Gartrell NK. Sex differences in medical student mental health. Am J Psychiatry 1981;138:1346-1351.

Lurie N, Rank B, et al. How do house officers spend their nights? N Engl J Med 1989;320:1673-1677.

Mawardi B. Satisfaction, dissatisfaction and causes of stress in medical practice. JAMA 1979;241:1483-1486.

McCall TB. The Libby Zion case. N Engl J Med 1988;318:771-778.

McCall TB. No turning back: A blueprint for residency reform. JAMA 1989;261: 909-910.

McCue JD. The effects of stress on physicians and their medical practice. N Engl J Med 1982;306(8):458-476.

McCue J. The distress of internship. N Engl J Med 1985;312:449-452.

McKegney CP. Medical education: A neglectful and abusive family system. Fam Med 1989;21:452-457.

Murphy M. Stress management classes as health promotion tool. A Canadian Nurse, June 1981, pp 29-31.

Myers MF. Doctor's Marriages. Plenum Press, New York, 1988, p. 34.

Nixon P. The human function curve: With special reference to: Cardiovascular disorders. Practitioner 1976;935:217,765,935.

Page L. Survey: Female residents face harassment, discrimination. Am Med News, December 8, 1989, p. 10.

Regelson W. Physician "burnout". In Professional Burnout in Medicine and the Helping Professions, Wessels DT, Jr., Kutscher AH, Seeland IB, et al, eds., Haworth Press, New York, 1989.

Reuben DB, Novack DH, Watchel TJ, Wartman SA. A comprehensive support system for reducing housestaff distress. Psychosomatics 1984;25:815-820.

Sandson J. Moonlighting medical students. N Engl J Med 1985;312:864.

Scadron A, Witte M, Axelrod M, et al. Attitudes toward women physicians in medical academia. JAMA 1981;247(20):2803-2807.

Schwartz AF et al. Levels and causes of stress among residents. J Med Educ 1987;62:744-753.

Selder FE, Paustian A. Burnout: Absence of vision. In Professional Burnout in Medicine and the Helping Professions, Wessels DT, Jr., Kutscher AH, Seelang IB, et al, eds., Haworth Press, New York, 1989.

Selye H. The stress of life. McGraw-Hill Book Co., NY, 1976.

Smith JW, Denny WF, Witzke DB. Emotional impairment in internal medicine housestaff. JAMA 1986;255:1155-1158.

Spears B. A time management system for preventing physician impairment. J Fam Pract 1981;13:175-180.

Spiegel DA, Smolen RC, Hopfensperger KA. Interpersonal stress in medical education: Correlates for men and women students. J Am Med Wom Assoc 1987;42(1):19-21.

Spiegel DA, Smolen RC, Jonas CK. As examination of the relationship among interpersonal stress, morale and academic performance in male and female medical students. Soc Sci Med 1986;23:1157-1161.

Storer JS, Floyd HH, et al. Effects of sleep deprivation on cognitive ability and skill of pediatric residents. Acad Med 1989;64:29-31.

Tokarz P. Promoting well-being through life planning. The Impaired Physician, Scientific Assembly, American Academy of Family Physicians, 1981.

Wagner M. Swingshift encephalopathy. Acad Med 1989;64:584.

Wallis C. Stress--Can we cope? Time, June 6, 1983.

Wessells DT, Jr., Kutscher AH, Seeland IR, et al, eds. Professional burnout in medicine and the helping professions. Haworth Press, NY, 1989.

Woods SM, Natterson J, Silverman J. Medical students' disease: Hypochondriasis in medical education. J Med Educ 1966;41:785-790.

Young EH. Relationship of residents' emotional problems, coping behaviors, and gender. J Med Educ 1987;62:642-650.

Zonderman AB, Costa PT, McCrae RR. Depression as a risk for cancer morbidity and mortality in a nationally representative sample. JAMA 1989;262(9):1191-1196.

"As a minority female physician at a university-based residency program, I am aware of my role as a pioneer. There are a few women medical faculty. The issues relative to being a female are more visible than those relative to race. Doors open slowly, with moderate effort."

Dr. Alica D. Monroe
Faculty Position-Family Practice
Married, Three School-age Children

9
Female Physician Stress

In one survey, 66% of women physicians indicated that they had had at least one very difficult period in their lives and felt that they were frequently "skating on thin ice" (Cartwright). This is indicative of a relatively high level of stress. The practicing women physicians in Cohen's study (1988) cited the following as the greatest detractors to career development: unable to work long hours without distraction (cited by 20% of the women), lack of female role model (19%), lack of satisfactory household help (12%), lack of confidence in personal competence (11%), lack of satisfactory child care (11%), lack of sponsors and/or mentors (9%), and unable to relocate to advance career (10%). Men cited these areas much less often.

The three major sources of unique stress for women physicians are their minority status/prejudice, lack of role models/mentors/sponsors, and role strain. All are interrelated. Since women physicians are a minority, they lack sufficient role models, which makes it more difficult for them to function well with role strain.

Minority Status/Prejudice/Discrimination

When Carole Lopate's book Women in Medicine was first published in 1969, a male physician reviewer made several negative comments: "unless the girl agrees to take vows of celibacy on entering medical school, it is reasonable to conclude that she should be factored out." (Lurie) He surmised the woman physician who was married and/or a mother would not work. He also believed there was unlikely to be any demand for women physicians since female patients would find it less threatening to their ego to reveal their bodily imperfections to a male than a female! Further, he insinuated that the female's 'well-known proclivity to gossip' would be detrimental to patient confidentiality. His prejudices are quite evident to us today.

One female surgery chief resident relates a story where she, with her entourage of junior residents, all male, walked into a room to greet an elderly male patient lying in bed. His comment to the female chief was,

"You stay with these smart men here, young lady. They'll teach you a lot."
(Vital Signs)

An example of double prejudice is that of a black female obstetrician.
During a severe storm, she was asked by another obstetrician to attend a
delivery because he could not get to the hospital. When she entered the
room to approach the patient, the patient said, "What is this place, Grand
Central Station? First, the orderlies, then the nurse and now the maid."
(Vital Signs)

Every female physician has a repertoire of similar experiences where she
has been mistaken for the nurse, family member, daughter and/or the least
experienced on the medical team. Many patients will ask female physicians
for the bedpan, new icewater or other items, for which they would not
think of asking male physicians. It is not uncommon for pharmacists to
question a woman's right to prescribe over the phone, whereas they would
not so question a man.

There are various ways to explain these types of prejudices; this section
will compare the prejudice faced by women as physicians to those of other
types of minorities in majority cultures, or the out-group as compared to
the in-group. Much of this is based on "The Tale of O," a filmstrip, and
the work of Kanter (1977).

The Process of Assimilation The advancement of women in medicine and
the prejudices that they face can be compared to what is known about the
advancement and assimilation of other minorities into groups. The first
step in the process is the introduction of the first minority. This individual
and the first few others that are added become labeled as 'test cases.' The
magnifying glass is focused on these individuals and any mistakes or
insecurities cannot be hidden. The test person is a novelty. Everything the
person says or does is remembered. This constant scrutiny often leads to
the burden of feeling that every action will affect all of the same type of
minority who follow. Women physicians often believe that, as with any
other minority group, they must be especially good and careful, lest any
shortcomings be chalked up to their sex rather than treated as an
individual matter (Rapoport).

Once the test case has been in the group and additional members of
the minority are added, their status changes to that of an 'exceptional
minority'. They continue to be viewed as minorities, but are placed into
an identifiable slot with which the accepting group will be comfortable.
This 'slot' or niche carries with it identifiable prejudice and biased
behaviors. There are greater differences between the minority group and
majority group than within the minority group (see also Park) Deviations
by minority members from majority group expectations are not well

tolerated by majority members. Members of the minority continue to be closely scrutinized, and prejudice based on the status of the minority persists.

Only when the group becomes close to half of the total group (or when their numbers are sufficiently large and a new type of minority is introduced), is there a balance reached where the differences within the minority group are greater than the difference between the minority and majority group. When this occurs there is true assimilation and prejudice tends to be minimal.

These steps in the process of assimilation result at least partially from the psychology of the in-group (majority) versus the out-group (minority). (See the seminal work of Allport 1958.) As the in-group has more contact with the out-group, prejudice tends to decrease--the majority finds out that many of their prejudices and generalizations do not hold. Greater numbers of the minority group result in more contact and therefore decrease prejudice.

The Test Case Many woman speak of the loneliness of being selected for special attention because of their sex (as the test case) and how unreasonable it is to represent a whole class of persons every day. The first women in medical school felt that they could never simply be themselves, but were being tested and watched constantly (Spiro). Each day the decision as to whether women would be admitted to the medical school the next year could rest on their behavior. This process can be self-fulfilling, resulting in a passive, insecure professional woman (Batt).

Southgate (1975) has discussed how the singularity of the test case forced women physicians to cope with isolation and lack of companionship. A woman in medical school in the 1950s was frequently reminded that she was displacing a man for similar training. The insinuation was that she would be depriving our culture of the badly needed (male) physician. Women students thus felt indebtedness that they would never be able to pay back. Marriage/motherhood and medicine were considered a contradiction. Nuns usually had a better chance of getting into medical school for this reason, and attractive women had the most difficulty entering (Southgate). Women entering medical school 15 to 25 years ago were thus placed in the position of apologizing and feeling like they had to succeed at any cost. This resulted in unrealistic standards for how they should perform (Southgate).

It must be noted that there are also some perceived advantages to being a test case. As a novelty, the first woman or women may well receive special attention and benefits. Perhaps the organization would like to have one woman, just to show that they are not 'prejudiced' or do not 'discriminate.' Test case women often feel they have attained their position, power, or friendliness with men solely because they are different and obvious, regardless of their capabilities. There may be some truth to this, which makes it all the more difficult for women to assess their true self-worth. In actuality, many of these women are overqualified, rather than underqualified for their positions. The overall effect, however, is that some 'test case' women resist the entrance of other women who threaten their privileged position. This is unfortunate because it is at least partially a lack of confidence and certainly a result of prejudice that makes these women feel that it is not their capabilities but uniqueness that has given them privilege. These women often fail to understand that having more women in the same organization or field would decrease the overall prejudices, and provide all women with greater gain.

Exceptional Minority Status and Prejudice As the numbers of the minority increase modestly, a different set of expectations and behaviors are exhibited. Prejudice, labeling and stereotyping are common when the members of the minority have reached numbers sufficient to make them an 'exceptional minority.' Prejudice is the distortion of perception and experience based on preconceived expectations and prejudged beliefs. I.e., people see things the way they want to see them and the way they think they should be. Labeling and stereotyping are related forms of prejudice.

Labeling is a stereotyping method of prejudice against women in which descriptive or identifying terminology is used in a biased fashion for women as compared to men. For example, an intelligent person is smart, if male, but helpful, if female. Innovative is original in men and pushy in women. An insistent personality is persistent if male and hysterical if female. Men are assertive, women are aggressive. This differential labeling distorts the impact of behavior which is actually identical (Batt). Thus, the adverse labeling of the qualities of leadership that are needed for advancement in medicine make the woman undesirable. It is no wonder that women professionals, including women physicians, lack the confidence and self-assertion to take leadership roles.

Typically, the stereotypes that women assume or are assumed to follow can be divided into the following:

1. The Helper -- a good listener, "gopher" and coffee maker (The Tale of "O").
2. The Sex Object -- ultrafeminine, not taken seriously (The Tale of "O").

3. The Mascot or Cheerleader -- young, lively, and enthusiastic, they always make the men around them feel better (The Tale of "O").
4. The Militant -- rebellious against the prejudice (The Tale of "O").
5. One of the Boys -- looks, works and acts like one of the group (Pfeiffer, Konanc).
6. The Sexless Woman -- denounces all differences between masculine and feminine perspectives (Potter).
7. The Mother -- a caretaker who cooks, cleans, listens and cares for the men.

One of the problems is that none of these stereotypes, with the possible exception of "one of the boys," emphasizes the performance and risk-taking necessary for advancement in the organization. The sex role socialization of women has generally taught them to seek male approval, avoid conflict and anger, and, as a result, women have little preparation for advancement to positions of authority and power (Potter).

Women in medicine have been perceived as "violating" the existing group the same way any minority violates the majority and are subject to stereotyping and prejudice from male colleagues (Potter). Overt discrimination occurs when teachers bait and tease women students (Campbell). Faculty may stereotype women students as "too masculine," "non-motherly," "certainly not a proper girlfriend," or "too pretty to be a medical student." (Johnson, Scott, Cartwright)

Bias exists to a far greater degree than most physicians would care to think. Women students continue to be harassed in the classroom because of their sex and pay the price for this in anger and damage to their self-esteem (Roeske). They also face the hazing typically given to all medical students. In a way, they receive double hazing. If a woman seeks any special favors or becomes aggressive, she can expect negative reactions from the group (Angell). This is consistent with "exceptional minority" status--as long as women accept their place, it is okay; if a woman steps out of bounds, the majority becomes angry and condemns the individual and the minority group.

Until the last 15 years, there were often no arrangements for women to sleep in the hospital while they were on call (Campbell). Many women were forced to sleep wherever there was an unoccupied bed in the hospital. Locker rooms continue to this day to be marked "doctors" and "nurses." The male doctors forget that the dictaphones, the coffee and a great deal of medical discussion are held in the 'doctor's' locker room.

Some of women's complaints of prejudice are seen by male physician counterparts as somewhat less than "sisterly." These same male physicians do not comprehend why this bothers women, or, as they see it, why women do not want to stick with other women, i.e., the nurses, their "sisters." The resistance to making adequate provisions for women once they are in school and training remains a significant form of prejudice encountered by women.

A more subtle type of prejudice occurs in male-female interactions in the workplace, including the hospital. Female behavior, such as wearing makeup and attractive clothing, may lead to the notorious "pass." Because of the social structure of medical institutions, women on lower levels of training tend to be preyed upon by men in higher positions, who use their authority to press for sexual favors. Women in medicine talk of times when male doctors (usually superiors), coming into call rooms or otherwise, approach women sexually, creating confusion and anger.

Prejudice, stereotyping and labeling result in insecurity and a lack of confidence on the part of the minority, which in turn has other consequences. Insecurity on the part of women physicians can be transferred to others, raising questions in the minds of other physicians or patients about their competence or abilities. Prejudice against women physicians can be and is evidenced by other women physicians, other women health care providers and by patients. Many women physicians themselves are prejudiced toward their younger peers, either fearing they themselves will lose the positive aspects of their singularity, or believing the younger women are not competent, just as they are unsure of their own competence. Other women health care providers may have negative attitudes about women physicians --a woman physician is evidence that a woman can make it and yet they themselves did not pursue medical school because of built-in biases and insecurity. For them, women physicians may represent their own failures. Female as well as male patients may also be prejudiced against women physicians, preferring male physicians for various reasons.

In one study (Konanc), women physicians encountered prejudice at all levels of medical school. Verbal comments from professors, housestaff and male peers ranged from direct putdowns to indirect insinuations of failure. A common problem noted is 'spotlighting,' where the minority is asked 80% of the questions. Sometimes women students tell each other that one needs to be sure that there will be at least one other woman on the same rotation at the same time in order to prevent this type of harassment. On rotations, it would appear that a woman cannot win. If she is too quiet and passive, she is graded down, or, if she is too aggressive, graded down. The result is the same. Comments in evaluations are often about a woman's personality rather than skills (Konanc). Instances of subtle discrimination were frequently cited by support group members (Konanc).

One example was the invisible woman excluded from sports discussions, yet the object of sexual wisecracks and heterosexual flirtations (Konanc, Campbell). About half of the women in one study (Konanc) believed the prejudices were not difficult to handle. Whether or not the prejudice was acknowledged, minimized or handled smoothly, it was indeed a common experience for women medical students, and may well have a subtle impact on the women's long-term confidence and ability to assert themselves in the medical world.

Full Assimilation Full assimilation for women physicians will take some time. The numbers of women in medicine do not yet approach the fifty percent mark, nor will they for many years to come. With the influx of women into medical schools, complaints of sexism have greatly diminished, consistent with incorporation of a minority group (women) into the majority group (men). The sheer number of women in medical school today makes it possible for women to feel more comfortable than they once did, yet real attitudinal change from the current structure will not come for a period of years. Present harmful behavior patterns should continue to be discouraged to make life more tolerable for the female physician (Howell). As influx of women approaching the numbers necessary for full assimilation are first noted in the training years, women will face less prejudice in their years in medical school prior to noting a decrease in the practice years. Only when prejudice has been defeated will women be equal to men in medicine.

Lorber (1984) argues that full assimilation is unlikely to occur on the basis of numbers alone. She believes that the discrimination against women is often subtle, but pervasive. White men in power tend to sponsor and support people like themselves, i.e, other white men, whom they inherently believe they can trust more. Furthermore, she argues that women must band together to fight for women's rights, for otherwise, even with 50% of physicians being of the female sex, they will net little power.

Lack of Role Models/Mentors/Sponsors

Many men and some women physicians do not understand the basic need for women to have female role models. Women without role models are in a psychological quandary (Dowling). They do not know which parent to be like or how to handle their situation. Who should the woman identify with? This confusion has been termed "gender panic" (Dowling).

The female medical student may wonder how to maintain her identity as a woman and be a physician. There are relatively few women in prominent faculty and administrative positions to serve as role models or mentors. Also, the women who are visible in medicine present only one aspect of the total arrangement of possible lifestyles (Nadelson). With few female models, women physicians may style themselves in terms of the male image, although many young professional women no longer see the model of masculinity as viable. At the present time, women physicians along with other women professionals, are striving to create a new image of femininity that will encompass a multitude of potentials and possibilities of total human beings instead of becoming 'one of the boys' (Cartwright).

The traditional female concept of being helpless and dependent is of little value in medical school where leadership and assertiveness are expected (Batt). Some women medical students resolve this particular stress by adopting a competitive-aggressive stance. Another subgroup silently denies any problems whatsoever by failing to perceive any negative attitudes. A woman who does not become one of the boys often feels isolated and lonely because she is not accepted in the group. At times of stress, she may receive less support from her male classmates (Stephen). These women appear passive, compliant and noncompetitive which seems to fit the more traditional female identity. In spite of stresses, some women claim not to experience conflict with the issue of female identity (Pfeiffer, Konanc).

Since medicine is a male-dominated field, many of the assumptions, values and expectations are men's. Thus, the image of the ideal physician is more in terms of the male physician than the female one. Traditionally, this has meant a life-long commitment and involvement in medicine and has demanded nothing less from physicians than selfless dedication to others. This is difficult for even the most committed of men. Also, physicians' wives have been willing to shoulder the day-to-day problems in the marriage and the family, thus enabling her husband to be totally committed to the profession. This possibility has essentially not existed for women physicians. The field of medicine has not felt it necessary to change its expectations of the ideal physician because of the multiple and different commitments women bring to the medical career (Cartwright).

Without the necessary role models, these issues are more difficult to approach. Women often do not actively seek out or recognize directly their role models, but the effect is subtle. Women physicians who graduated from McMaster University in retrospect believe their career development was inhibited by the lack of role models (Cohen); 19% of women in practice cited the lack of a same sex role model as an inhibitor to career development, whereas only 1% of men did so. Similarly, academic women internists found it difficult to find role models, although two-thirds had had a mentor during their training (Levinson). The presence of other women who have 'made it', who have dealt effectively with being a woman physician, who are confident, secure and professional, creates a lasting impression and provides a basis for the individual's own sense of worth and coping strategies. Thus, the nonavailability of role models creates and additional stress for women physicians.

Furthermore, sponsors who help to provide key support at different times in the career enhance career development. Sponsors tend to help individuals who are similar to them, i.e., the same sex and race. As Lorber (1984) points out, women often lack key advocates in the form on sponsors, partially because of the lack of women in the position to do so. Women physicians in practice in Cohen's study noted the lack of sponsors and/or mentors 9% of the time, with men doing so 2% of the time.

Role Strain

Role strain for the female physician is the conflict that results from having to choose between the multiple demands placed on her by her profession and those that arise from her obligations as a mother, a wife, and a person in her own right (Pfeiffer). Continued societal expectations that women have the major responsibility for the home and children, whether or not they have a full-time career, have created much of the role strain. Caring for a family and pursuing a full-time career is physically and emotionally taxing (Baucum-Copeland) and family responsibilities are listed by women physicians as a detraction from career development moreso than by men physicians (Cohen). The greatest stress perceived as prominent guilt and anxiety appears to be related to the role of mother (Johnson).

In their book Gender and Stress, Barnett et al (1987) conclude that women are inherently more stressed than men, primarily because of the role of mother, which has high demands and is low in control, in contrast to the role of father which is traditionally low in demands and high in control. They go on to say, "Indeed, the price of being a fully socialized female in our culture may be a predisposition to feelings of lack of control and ultimately to depression" (Barnett, p. 358). Working or marriage had less to do with overall well-being than the negative effect of being a mother, particularly a mother of pre-school or numerous children (Barnett, p. 132). However, a more recent 18 year follow-up study (Kotler) found to impact on mortality of employment, having children, or having children in the home, except perhaps for single working women with children in the home. In fact Kotler (1989) notes that mortality was lowest for working married women with a least one child in the home and highest for unemployed single women with no child in the home and concludes that a multiplicity of roles does not appear to worsen mortality.

Even more problematic is the expectation that mothering is natural, and thus should engender neither stress nor expressions of stress (Barnett, p. 133). According to Aneshensel (1987), interrole conflict is greater when family role demands are extreme or inflexible or commitment to work is strong.

Similarly, in comparison to male physicians, women physicians experience more role strain in the areas of childcare, household responsibilities and marriage commitments (Cohen). At the same time, women indicate very little stress related to income, location of practice, spouse's occupation or number of children (Kaplan). In one study (Cartwright), 51% of female physicians felt some intermittent role strain and 20% experienced much strain. Only a third had achieved what they felt to be harmonious integration of their roles. The two variables that related negatively to role harmony were the number of children and the women's age, i.e., the more children or the older the woman physician, the greater the role strain.

Most women and physicians combine family, career and the experience of pregnancy at some time during their medical careers (Bonar). The juggling act that this requires is often most intense in the woman's 30s. This is a time when career development is most rapid for men, but the woman physician is likely to be in the midst of raising her young children as well as developing her career (Angell). It is difficult for the woman physician not to compare herself and her career development with that of her counterparts in the male world.

In one study 30% of women physicians had no domestic help (Heins 1977). Seventy-six percent of the respondents did all the cooking, shopping, childcare and money management for the household. Even in dual-career marriages, women continue to be responsible for the children, regardless of their level of professional commitment (Eisenberg). The responsibilities for household work is compounded by the unavailability of qualified household help or by the available help being unskilled in childcare. Frequently the available childcare is from a different economic or educational class and has different childbearing practices as viewed by the physician (Heins 1982).

Being a spouse is more stressful for women than men. In terms of health, just being married is beneficial to men, whereas for employed women, equity and supportiveness of the spouse are particularly important (Belle). Husbands confide more in wives than vice versa; husbands generally feel more support from their spouses than wives do (Belle).

Summary

Female physicians are definitely stressed, probably moreso when they are mothers and minorities within their profession. However, literature on women in general suggest that, in spite of greater stressors, women live longer than men, perhaps because they are emotionally more expressive (Barnett, p. 357). Employment is positively associated with improved health for women and the more high-power the career the more health advantage there is (Barnett p. 134). Thus, when the stresses are well controlled, women physicians should have a major advantage in well-being over other women. Women physicians overall seem to have a high life satisfaction (Ducker, Cartwright 1978).

References

Allport GW. The nature of prejudice, Second Edition. Garden City, New York, Doubleday Anchor Books, 1958.

Aneshensel CS, Pearlin LI. Structural contexts of sex differences in stress. In Gender & Stress, Barnett RC, Beiner L, Baruch GK, eds. The Free Press, Macmillan, Inc., New York, 1987.

Angell M. Juggling a personal and professional life. J Am Med Wom Assoc 1982;37(3):64-68.

Barnett RC, Beiner L, Baruch GK, eds. Gender & Stress. The Free Press, Macmillan, Inc., New York, 1987.

Batt R. Creating a professional identity. Am J Psychoanalysis 1972;32(2):156-162.

Baucum-Copeland M, et al. Pregnant resident: Career conflict. J Am Med Wom Assoc 1983;38(4):103-105.

Bonar J, Watson J, et al. Sex differences in career and family plans of medical students. J Am Med Wom Assoc 1982;37(11):300-303.

Campbell MA. Why would a girl go into medicine? The Feminist Press, New York, 1973.

Cartwright L. Career satisfaction and role harmony in a sample of young women physicians. J Voc Beh 1978;12184-12196.

Cohen M, Woodward CA, Ferrier BM. Factors influencing career development: Do men and women differ? J Am Med Wom Assoc 1988;43(5):142-154.

Dowling C. Cinderella Complex. Simon & Schuster New York, New York, 1981.

Ducker DG. Life satisfactions for women physicians. J Am Med Wom Assoc 1987;42:57-59.

Eisenberg C. Women as physicians. J Med Educ 1983;58:534-541.

Grundy B. Career roles in medicine. A paper presented at the American Psychological Association, Hawaii 1972.

Heins M. Medicine and motherhood. JAMA 1982;249(2):209-210.

Heins M, Smock S, et al. A profile of the woman physician. J Am Med Wom Assoc 1977;32(11):421-427.

Howell M. What medical schools teach you about women. N Engl J Med 1974;291 (6):304-307.

Johnson C, Johnson F. Attitudes toward parenting in dual-career families. Am J Psychiatry 1977;134:4.

Kaplan H. Women physicians--The more effective recruitment and utilization of their talents and their resistance to it. The Woman Physician September 1970;25:9.

Konanc J. What support groups for women medical students do: A retrospective inquiry. J Am Med Wom Assoc 1979;34:282.

Kotler P, Wingard DL. The effect of occupational, marital and parental roles on mortality: The Alameda County study. Am J Public Health 1989;79:607-612.

Levinson W, Tolle SW, Lewis C. Women in academic medicine: Combining career and family. N Engl J Med 1989;321(22):1511-1517.

Lopate C. Women in Medicine. Johns Hopkins Press for The Josiah Macy, Jr. Foundation, 1968.

Lorber J. Women physicians: Careers, status, and power. Tavistock Publications, New York, 1984.

Luri A. A matter of perspective. Medical Opinion and Review 1979;45(5):39-40.

Nadelson C, Notman M. The woman physician. J Med Educ 1972;47:176-184.

Nadelson T, Isenberg L. Successful professional women: On being married to one. Am J Psychiatry 1977;134:10.

Park B, Rothbart M. Perception of out-group homogeneity and levels of social categorization: Memory for the subordinate attributes of in-group and out-group members. J Personality & Social Psychology 1982;42(6):1051-1068.

Pfeiffer RF. Early adult development in the medical student. Mayo Clin Proc 1983;58:127-134.

Potter RL. Resident, woman, wife, mother: Issues for women in training. J Am Med Wom Assoc 1983;38:4.

Rapoport R, Rapoport R. Further considerations on a dual-career family. Human Relations 1971;24(6):519-533.

Roeske N, Lake K. Role models for women medical students. J Med Educ 1977;52:459-466.

Southgate M. Remembrance of things (hopefully) past. JAMA 1975;232(13): 1331-1332.

Spears B. A time management system for preventing physician impairment. J Fam Pract 1981;13:175-180.

Spiro H. Myths and mirths--Women in medicine N Engl J Med 1977;53:459-466.

Stephen B. What's the best time to have a baby? Redbook, February 1983;40-45.

The Tale of "O"--On being different. Produced by Goodmeasure, Inc. Cambridge, Massachusetts, 1979.

Vital Signs. Medica: Women Practicing Medicine, New York, Medica Publishers, Fall 1983, p 31.

Free to Cry

"I believe crying is healthy. I use it to reduce stress or to give expression to my deepest feelings; but, primarily, I use it to feel the pain of my patients and to convey to them the understanding of my heart. Being a woman allows me to cry as a physician. I am not bound by society's rules but, rather, given the privilege of tears because I am of a female nature. When I was a brand new intern, spending my first week on the medical wards, I remember vividly one particular morning. I had been up all night on call and had admitted a number of patients. I felt neither in control nor able to handle the medical task before me. That morning on rounds with one of the attendings, I began crying openly when presenting one of the patients. My tears were born of fatigue, fear of failure, frustration and disenchantment with medicine. I will never forget the attending's response. He put his arm around me, comforted me and told me that things would get better. I have often wondered since then, would he have been this kind to one of my male colleagues? At worst, I am sure he considered this display of emotion the outburst of a fragile female; at best, he probably remembered his own early training and the significant emotion this brings. Tears do not come so easily to most men in the medical profession. Too often they have been raised and regulated out of this free display of emotion, this release of tension, this deepest communication with those who are suffering. Perhaps, it is one of the responsibilities of women in medicine to allow ourselves to use tears in such ways and to help our male colleagues to rediscover this freeing form of emotion."

Ellen Brubeck, M.D.
Family Physician
Married, Mother
Mid-Career

10
Physician Marriages and Dual Career Couples

Current statistics indicate that three-quarters of female physicians marry (see chapter 6 on Mental Health). About 85% of these will marry another professional, and about 50% marry other physicians. According to Parker and Jones (1981), a female physician who marries another professional will judge her professional existence more satisfactory than if she were married to a nonprofessional. Thus over half of women physicians have dual career marriages and many have dual-doctor marriages.

Physician Marriages

There is some question as to whether or not the medical personality lends itself to being a poor marriage partner (Fine). The adjectives usually used to describe the medical personality are bright and energetic, coupled with goal oriented, detached and dedicated to work. These attributes may result in a lack of committed time to anything other than work and the spouses of physicians tend to believe they are 'living alone yet with someone.' The physician is "married to his/her career." (Fine, Gerber)

On the other hand, Doherty and Burge (1989) found that there is some evidence that divorce may actually be less common among physicians than other employed professional male and females (see also chapter 6 on Mental Health). Physicians marry later in life, which may help explain the lower divorce rate.

For both the male and female physician, marriage introduces two incompatible elements. Marriage is supposed to provide support, but creates a web of responsibility to which the physician may be less than committed (Gabbard 1987). Early in the medical marriage both spouses may view as temporary the difficulty of blending personal and professional lives. Accepting delayed gratification is a central component in the compulsive personality of the physician. During medical school and residency, studies and supervisors are easily targeted as the 'cause' of marital problems. But the training does end, and the realization that the spouse will not change comes slowly. The psychology of postponement ultimately proves to be the psychology of avoidance. The avoidance grows directly out of the compulsive personality traits of most physicians and their preference (often subconscious) for work over family life (Gabbard and Menninger 1989).

Gabbard and Menninger (1988) found that both physicians and spouses ranked the same issues as sources of conflict in the medical marriage. Both ranked "lack of time for fun, family and self" as the leading source of conflict.   Physicians see "time away from home at work" as a much more important source of conflict than their spouses. Spouses considered lack of intimacy as a much more serious problem than did the physicians. This is not surprising since over 90% of the spouses in this survey were female and intimacy is a central concern for women.

Gabbard feels that lack of time serves as a convenient excuse for most couples. He feels that this complaint serves the function of attributing conflicts in the marriage to factors outside of marriage. Actual conflicts arise around differences in three areas: the need for intimacy (spouse needs more than physician), perceptions of problems in the relationship, and communication styles (females prefer talking, males prefer sex) (Scheier).

Though the characteristics of the female spouse of the male physician are changing, still, the largest profession recorded by this group is "homemaker." In the study done by Nadelson (1979) at Harvard over a 10-year period, she found that over 90% of the male physicians had a spouse who stayed at home. In a study of over 3,000 family physicians done by Ogle et al (1986), 74% of the husbands of female family physicians had earned graduate degrees as compared to 30% of the wives of the male physicians. For males in this study, 2/3 of the spouses were not employed outside the home. Only 13% were employed full-time. In contrast, 98.9% of the spouses of female physicians were employed full time. Wives of male physicians were less likely to be working outside of the home if there were small children in the family.   The likelihood of outside work decreased with each additional child. These trends were not present in the marriages of female physicians.   Husbands were highly likely to be employed regardless of the number of children.

Female Physician Marriages

"Most people look upon marriage as a potential support to male physicians, but see marriage as a potential burden for most female physicians." (Vincent) In one study, women physicians over age 45 scored their husbands as being somewhat unsupportive and against their careers (Parker). Nearly twice the percentage of women physicians as compared to men expect to interrupt their careers to accommodate a spouse's career

(Kaplan). Conversely, some theorize being married is a powerful, positive factor for men physicians and helps them buffer against many problems, including psychiatric disorders (Eisenberg). Men experience lower rates of depression and are healthier than single, separated or divorced men (Eisenberg; Cleary). Alternatively, marriage does not have a protective effect on health for women (Cleary).

The husband who is supportive of the woman pursuing a medical career will tend to be supportive of her in general and more helpful with domestic and parental responsibilities. If the female physician has a supportive husband, she will be more satisfied in her medical practice and less likely to work reduced hours (Parker). In general, a supportive husband, rather than just a husband, is important to the emotional health of the employed woman (Belle), i.e., the quality of the marriage is the key (Wethington). For mothers, "the health advantage . . . of being employed was negated if their husband did not participate in child care." (Barnett p. 136) Thus, the choice of a husband may be one of the most significant choices a woman physician can make.

Women physicians expect equal sharing of child care and household responsibilities, while men expect to contribute less than their wives to these tasks (Kaplan). However, fathers who care more for children in the mother's absence rate their marriages more poorly (Barnett p. 137). Despite high expectations, women continue to bear the major responsibilities for the family and home (Heins). If male partners are helpful in the home, they are often self-congratulatory and awarded accolades for the effort (Nadelson 1977), but may suffer more depression (Barnett p. 139). Hopefully, the inequality is changing, at least modestly. There seems to be some indication that men are diminishing their intense career commitment and increasing their level of family involvement, while women appear to be going in the opposite direction (Eisenberg). This is also suggested by the convergence in female and male physicians' productivity (see chapter 4 on Productivity). Lorber (1982) also found that patterns were changing in couples under 40 years of age. Decisions appeared to be more mutual and both spouses appeared to value a spouse who could understand their professional problems. Competition between the two individuals did not appear to be a major problem, but some of these couples had difficulty separating their professional identities.

Meyers (1984) claims that some women who study medicine have not grown up with a comfortable sense of themselves as being appealing or attractive to men. For these women, their scholastic achievement and ambition alone set them apart from peers of both sexes. The woman doctor who is unsure of herself as a woman will feel inferior in a marriage. She may be uncomfortable asserting herself for fear of loosing her spouse.

Meyers also believes that guilt is always present in women doctors with marital problems. He does not mean the normal guilt experienced by all perfectionistic females, but an incapacitating guilt exemplified by anxiety attacks and depressive symptomatology. The woman physician feels that if she just worked a little harder she alone should be able to correct the problems in the marriage.

One stressor unique to women physicians is that they constantly give of themselves both at home and at the office.   When work is done, a married female physician arrives home and is required by her family and herself to be a loving supportive wife and mother. In contrast, a man often arrives home to his major source of emotional support (his wife) and is not expected to be as nurturing. Clearly, as the primary nurturer, the woman is left with very little time or energy to nurture herself (McKay).

Dual-Career Marriages

Some doctors tend to be authoritarian and find it hard to be democratic and egalitarian in a dual-career marriage (Fine).   One of the most important costs of a dual-career marriage is the time lost to the companionship of the spouse.   This is a cost borne equally by both partners. Some believe that women may feel the impact more since they may be socialized into roles that are more expressive and thereby may feel a greater need for dependency and affectionate feedback for maintenance of their self esteem (Nadelson).

A second cost of the dual-career marriage may be the male spouse's ego identification. The male physician in a dual-career family may experience anxiety because he is not living up to his perceived expectation of his masculine role. He may be devalued by his colleagues, and perhaps by himself. The commonplace chores of domestic life challenge even the liberated husband's commitment to an egalitarian marriage (Nadelson).

A third cost may be sexual problems. One paper (Johnson) gives case descriptions of sexual problems arising in dual-career families primarily related to shifts in the balance of power between the two spouses. The authors attribute some of the low sex drive of their patients to sheer exhaustion secondary to the much heavier than average work and family schedules. In several of the cases discussed, sexual dysfunction was used as a manipulative factor by the husband to express hostility toward the wife. Another study (Potter) suggested that role strain in the two career medical student marriage leads to marital dysfunction with loss of sexual interest in the partner.

The physicians in Gabbard and Menninger's study (1988) lived up to the stereotype that portrayed them as being too busy and too tired to have sex. Frequency of sexual relations ranked high on the physicians list as a source of conflict in the marriage. The mean frequency of sexual relationships in this study was 1.6 times a week.

The Dual-Doctor Marriage

Dual-physician couples will become more of a phenomenon as more women enter medical school. At this time, the literature on two-physician couples is not extensive. While it is reasonable to assume that other professions are also demanding and that many of the problems encountered in dual-physician marriages are similar to those of the dual-professional families (Lorber), the dual-physician couple has the added demands of patient care and there are few role models available for them to follow (Heins 1977).

There are rewards, however, to being married to another physician. After the training period, physician husbands and wives seem to be colleagues and peers in practice and partners in continuing medical education (Lorber). The couples appear to become 'helpmates' for each other in career matters. The physician spouse is often turned to for advice and most dual-physician couples feel that the marriage is of benefit.

There are also unique problems for dual-doctor marriages. In addition to the burdens of patient care, there are problems in trying to match internships, residencies, fellowships and practices in the same location. With women now comprising a substantial number of graduating seniors, many physicians face the decision as to whether or not to match as a pair. One study shows that women medical students tend to 'marry down' and are often the stronger candidate in the match (Wineberger).

After finding training sites, there is a tendency in two-physician couples for one physician's career to dominate over the other. In the past, females have not experienced the same status or monetary rewards as males and have tended to devalue their career development and professionalism. Thus, the male's career in a dual-physician couple has tended to dominate. In virtually all cases studied previous to 1980 (Winter), the husband's career determined where the family lived and worked. A 1982 study by Kilpatrick reported that 35% of male candidates who were finalists for positions requiring relocation would not negotiate further unless their wives needs were also met. In fact, Eisenberg (1981) claims that the lower academic rank of women in professional careers stems from the geographic restriction imposed by a two-career household. This is supported by the fact that married women physicians lag behind single women physicians, as well as behind men, in academic advancements (Eisenberg), although there may also be other mitigating factors.

In addition to the problems on the professional front, there are those of the home environment. The question that appears most asked in every dual-doctor family is who will handle the administrative functions of the family such as staying home to deal with repair people, serving as a chauffeur to the children and chief cook. Dual-physician families tend to have their children in a compressed period with little interrupted work by the wife, accentuating the purely administrative hassles related to the family.

The Name of the Married Women Physician

When a woman marries, what should she do with her name? The male physician never has to concern himself with what he will be called when he is married, but marriage frequently brings about a personal crisis for women. Not assuming her partner's name is often perceived as a lack of commitment to the marriage and to the spouse's family. Dralle (1987) found in her study that 18% of married female physicians did not change there names, 64% took their husband's name. Another 16% used non-traditional variations of their names. She found that name changes had no connection to commitment to the marriage or satisfaction with their current name. She found, however, that women who entered medicine when their were fewer women tended to keep their original birth names (Dralle).

Thompson (1980) found the following problems tend to arise if a woman changes her name after she has established herself educationally:

1. If a woman changes her name with marriage and has written and published articles, she could have two or more entries in the Index Medicus.
2. Those who hyphenate find that the Library of Congress classifies a married woman under her husband's surname.
3. The old boy's network will never remember the recently married woman's new name.
4. If a physician's diploma is issued in her birth name and she later marries, she has to get her medical school diploma changed.
5. Patients may see diplomas and certificates in maiden names and raise questions about their doctor's credentials.
6. If the physician divorces and remarries, the coordination of the name problem becomes mind boggling.

Dealing with Two Careers

There has been little research done on the personality types that meet with success in a dual-career marriage. Apparently, the male needs to be nonthreatened by a career wife and secure in his masculine identity. He must be able to assume full responsibilities for household and childrearing as needed (Scott). The personalities of those individuals who were found to have the highest role harmony in dual-career couples were those associated with higher levels of confidence in all areas, higher levels of adjustment and relaxed nonjudgmental perspectives (Cartwright).

Time is simultaneously the most precious commodity and the greatest source of stress to any physician. To successfully accommodate a dual-career family, the couple must judiciously allocate time. Time will become more precious than money for them, and spending money to relieve the couple of chores may provide more time for both couple and family life. Allocation of time can be done by establishing priorities and goals, both long-term and short-term. Time management is very important. Scheduling should be done on a week to week basis so that each knows the activities of the other, but monthly and yearly activities must also be planned. This gives the couple time to schedule vacations and activities with and without the children. It may be necessary for both of the partners to limit work in order to have the number of nonwork hours needed to meet the goals of the couple. Some couples spend one weekend a month away from home just to nurture their relationship (Scott).

Gabbard and Menninger (1989) feel that the best way to save a physician-physician marriage is by preventive measures. Both physicians must realize that the marriage is an entity that requires the attention of both partners. It can be the main source of coping with the stress of medical practice, as well as the first potential casualty of that stress. After identifying the need for attention to the marriage, each spouse needs to verbalize his and her needs and expectations from the union. These authors recommend a mandatory time each day when spouses must sit down and discuss activities and plans. Attention must be made to the quality of the conversation also. The needs of each partner must be made explicit. Too many couples rely on mind reading. The final ingredient is the realization that no solution will be perfect. Most perfectionistic people (like doctors) often assume that there is a perfect arrangement for every problem. A more realistic view would be that it will be impossible to please everyone when trying to balance family and work life. The only solution is compromise. Each partner must make compromises in the direction of meeting the needs of the other person.

Heins et al (1982) suggest that husbands can help decrease some of the stress of the dual-career marriage by talking to their male colleagues about their home responsibilities. Children have been a forbidden topic of conversation at work for males and there seems to be a sense of shame when it is necessary to leave work to do something for the family. It will be impossible for medicine to be sensitive to the needs of the family if physicians tend to deny and not discuss these needs (Heins 1982). If men physicians shared their wife physician's concerns as wives and mothers, it might help legitimize certain issues that are currently shrugged off as merely women's issues (Angell).

Women physicians should not feel guilty about equality on the home front. The most important single factor in the career of a married woman physician is the man she marries. Women physicians need to stand back and let their husbands take some of the responsibility for household management (Angell). If a man begins to share household responsiblities and does a poor job, women tend to dive in and take over or criticize. This insures that the same effort will not be made again. Men must be allowed to assume responsibilities in their own way. If a man does not cook or clean in the exact manner that is expected of him, perhaps the expectation should be changed (Angell). Also, if such responsiblities are a new experience for him, he may improve with time as he learns how to better do the chores.

Social networks are also important to the dual-career couple. Socializing for dual-career couples often involves other dual-career couples, appropriately so since this helps to reduce the pressure for 'not being normal' and provides examples of how other couples manage. The couples may also have more in common. The wife's business associates appear to be drawn into the social circles more of dual-career families than in a conventional middle-class family becuase of the need for environmental support to sustain the dual-career pattern (Rapoport).

Impact of Rising Number of Dual Career Couples in Medicine

With what is known about physicians, several outcomes could be expected from the rising number of dual career couples in medicine. First, it could negatively affect the geographic distribution of physicians. It is generally easier for both individuals in a dual-career marriage to find satisfying work in large metropolitan environments. This could exaggerate the tendency of physicians to locate in urban rather than rural areas. Second, increasing dual-doctor couples could decrease the number of physicians, particularly women, belonging to professional organizations. Women may·be less likely to join organizations if their husbands belong. Third, overall productivity of physicians could decrease. As more physicians have higher-earner spouses, perhaps fewer will feel economic motivation to work long, hard hours. There may be more interest having sufficient home, leisure and family time rather than interest in work. Fourth, more systems to cater to dual-career couples will be developed. This may mean more family-options benefit packages, support systems at residency programs, etc.

Summary

Marriage and motherhood have many internal benefits for women physicians, but also create new and different stressors. While patently obvious, the choice of a husband is paramount, and the more supportive the husband, the better the mental health of the women physician. Marrying a husband with his own career, likewise adds additional constraints, particularly on the geographic moves sometimes needed for career advancement, time for leisure activities, and the complexity of management of the household. However, marrying another professional or physician increases income and may provide subtle additional support in the form of cross-fertilization of the individuals' careers. While considering all of these factors, specific attention must be made to the relationship of the couple to each other, to allow maximum personal fulfillment for both individuals.

References

Angell M. Juggling a personal and professional life. J Am Med Wom Assoc 1982;37(3):64-68. Barnett RC, Biener L, Baruch GK, eds. Gender & stress. The Free Press, Macmillan, Inc., New York, 1987.

Belle D. Gender differences in the social moderators of stress. In Gender & Stress, Barnett RC, Biener L, Baruch GK, eds., The Free Press, Macmillan, Inc., New York, 1987, p. 257-277. Cartwright L. Career satisfaction and role harmony in a sample of young women physicians. J Voc Beh 1978;12:184-196.

Cleary PD. Gender differences in stress-related disorders. In Gender & Stress, Barnett RC, Biener L, Baruch GK, Ed. The Free Press, New York, 1987, p. 39-72.

Doherty WJ, Burge SK. Divorce among physicians: Comparisons with other occupational groups. JAMA 1989;261(16):2374-2377.

Dralle PW. Women physicians' name choices at marriage. J Am Med Wom Assoc 1987;42(6):173-175.

Eisenberg L. Dystaff of Asculapius--The married woman as physician. J Am Med Wom Assoc 1981;36(2):84-88.

Fine C. Married to medicine: An intimate portrait of doctors' wives. Atheneum, New York, 1981.

Gabbard GO, Menninger RW, ed. Medical marriages. American Psychiatric Press, Washington, DC, 1988.

Gabbard GO, Menninger RW. The psychology of postponement in the medical marriage. JAMA 1989;261(16):2378-2381.

Gabbard GO, Menninger RW, Coyne L. Sources of conflict in the medical marriage. Am J Psychiatry 1987;144:567-572.

Gerber LA. Married to their careers. Tavistock Publications, New York, 1983.

Heins M. Medicine and Motherhood. JAMA 1982;249(2):209-210.

Heins M, Smock S, Martindale L. Current status of women physicians. Int J Women's Studies 1978;1(3):297-305.

Heins M, Smock S, Martindale L, et al. Comparison of productivity of women and men physicians. JAMA 1977;237(23):2514-2517.

Johnson F, Kaplan E, Tusel D. Sexual dysfunction in the two-career family. Med Asp Hum Sexuality 1979;13(9):7-17.

Kaplan H. Women physicians--The more effective recruitment and utilization of their talents and their resistance to it. The Woman Physician 1970;25(9):561-570.

Lorber J. How physicians' spouses influence each other's careers. J Am Med Wom Assoc 1982;37(1):21-26.

McKay MB, Alboszta M, Bingcang CC, et al. A stressor unique to married female physicians. Letter to the Editor. Am J Psychiatry 1986;143:114.

Myers MF. Overview: The female physician and her marriage. Am J Psychiatry 1984;141(11):1386-1391.

Myers MF. Doctors' marriages: A look at the problems and their solutions. Plenum Medical Book Company, New York, 1988.

Nadelson CC, Notman MT, Lowenstein P. The practice patterns, life styles, and stresses of women and men entering medicine: A follow-up study of Harvard medical School graduates from 1967 to 1977. J Am Med Wom Assos 1979;34(11):400-406.

Nadelson T, Eisenberg L. Successful professional women: On being married to one. Am J Psychiatry 1977;134:10.

Ogle KS, Henry RC, Durda K, Zivick JD. Gender-specific differences in family practice graduates. J Fam Pract 1986;23(4):357-360.

Parker G, Jones R. The doctor's husband. Br J Med Psych 1981;54:143-147.

Potter RL. Resident, woman, wife, mother: Issues for women in training. J Am Med Wom Assoc 1983;38(4):98-102.

Rapoport R, Rapoport R. Further considerations on a dual-career family. Human Relations 1971;24(6):519-533.

Scheier R. Patterns set in residency persist throughout marriage. Am Med News May 6 1988, p. 31.

Scott N. The balancing act. Universal Press Syndicate, Kansas City, 1978.

Thompson M. The professional name of women physicians: A plea for constancy. The New Physician April, 1980:p. 4-6.

Vincent MO. Female physicians as psychiatric patients. Can Psych Assoc J 1976;21(7):461-465.

Wethington E, McLeod JD, Kessler RC. The importance of life events for explaining sex differences in psychological distress. In Gender & Stress, Barnett RC, Biener

L, Baruch GK, eds., The Free Press, Macmillan, Inc., New York, 1987, p. 144-156.

Wineberger H, Oski F. Will a matchmaker kill the match? N Engl J Med 1982;307:320-321.

Winter R. Course helps future M.D.'s balance career, family life. American Medical News March 11, 1983, p. 26.

"The most stressful part of being a female physician is all the expectations I place on myself. To be the best doctor I can, the perfect wife, caring for aging parents, being active in my community, participating in medical politics, and still doing all the tasks of daily living to maintain myself and our household is overwhelming. I find it necessary to shift the priorities of these roles and most importantly, to make time to get away from them at regular intervals."

Marla Tobin, M.D.
Family Physician, Private Practice
Married 5 years, no children

11
Childbearing

Being a Physician can be Fulfilling. Being a Mother can be Fulfilling. Being a Physician and Mother can be...

It is generally accepted and expected that most women will have children, although this is less true than in the past. There is some acceptance for women, particularly professional women, to decide not to have children. The women physician must make a decision to have or not to have children. Does she want them? If so, when?

Women physicians as a group are career oriented: they must work very hard in order to receive the M.D. degree and they must work very hard to get board-certified. Once out in practice, the work continues. Medicine is, as discussed earlier, a profession, i.e., a field of endeavor with considerable expectations of dedication. Women physicians are devoted to and interested in their careers; can something else as similarly demanding as child-rearing be similarly important? Will it take them away from their career emotionally or physically? And, what will the men physicians think? Can she possibly do something not related to her career, miss that important meeting, or work fewer hours because the kids are sick, or, heaven forbid, just because she wants to be with them? What happens when pregnancy-related illness forces her to miss work? Will there be pressure from other co-workers? How will she personally accept the responsibilities? These questions arise again when the women physician decides to have additional children after the original decision was made and carried out.

Most women physicians do decide to have children, although there seems to be a discrepancy in the literature concerning the exact percentage of women physicians who are planning on having children. One study (Heins 1982) states that 85% of female students in medical schools plan to have children as compared to 90% of their male counterparts. Another study (Medica) claims that of the over 1,000 women physician surveyed in 1983, 30% were planning on remaining childless. Whatever the exact figure, a majority of women physicians will choose to have children. The number of children expected was 1.9 in 1970 (Kaplan), although the women in this study actually averaged 2.3 children. This is slightly greater than apparently was true in the past; Dykman (1953) found that slightly less than half of women physicians had children, and the women physicians who were married averaged 1.8 children. Of those women who had at least one child, the average was 2.4 children. A more recent figure appears to be 1.4 children per women physician (Sinal).

What About Me? What Should I Do?

In some ways there appears to be much in common between being a physician and being a mother. A physician is caring, dedicated and works long hours. The same is true of a mother. Both must set priorities. Both listen and help others to understand, to figure out and move ahead with their own lives. Both are important to society. Both are healers. Both feel guilty if they do not devote enough time or effort to their perceived duties. However one is a common role (i.e., motherhood) and one uncommon (i.e., a physician). The combination is somewhat more uncommon and the required juggling act can be difficult. The rewards of the two roles are different. One provides financial rewards; the other takes them away. One enables you to have nice material things; the other destroys them. One exalts you in public; in the other, you may be embarrassed to be in public if the child is crying or being destructive. Both are careers, however, and not simply 'jobs.'

The decision to have children is a very personal one. Each person must decide for her and himself. Clearly, the time and financial commitment inherent in childraising means forced prioritization once children are born. It becomes much more difficult to work a physician's 60 - 70 hours a week and still have time for oneself. One also never knows how she/he will personally react to the change in responsibilities--how much guilt will there be in combining career and parenthood? Kids are nonexistent ephemeral ideas in one's mind--that is, until they are born. Thus, how one will handle the responsibilities, whether one will enjoy or hate it, is unknown until the child is physically present. Even then, one never knows what the next stage of the child's life will bring. Thus, there will always be a certain amount of uncertainty; it is unavoidable.

Becoming pregnant involves physical and emotional risk. The fact that many people have had children and thoroughly enjoyed the experience may be reassuring, but does not guarantee that any one individual will react similarly, particularly a person who is different: the female physician has spent much of her life attaining her career goal. Having a family may always have seemed like a good idea, but what does it truly mean? Children can be the most fulfilling part of life, bringing great joy and satisfaction; they also can be very trying and emotionally distressing, both as young children and when older. Will I have enough time, energy and love to provide what I believe to be a good up-bringing? Yes, I always thought I could do anything (I proved that by becoming a physician), but can I accept a role that is fulfilling internally (for its own sake), as compared to externally (for the good of mankind)? A role whose reward comes more from direct interaction (children) than from the admiration of society and others (she's so great--she's a physician)?

If So, When?

If the answer is yes, then other decisions must be made. The choice of when to have a baby is a very individual matter. Each time period a woman physician might select is fraught with a variety of problems; each also has its unique benefits. The timing of childbearing a personal decision each woman will have to make, weighing the pros and cons for each time period in order to select the best alternative for her situation. However, even not deciding is a decision, because times marches on even while one is thinking.

Various Factors Go into the Timing of Having Children

The considerations are physiologic: how will my body handle it? will I be able to get pregnant? emotional: how will I feel? and practical: will there be the money? where can I get child care?

The time options for childbearing can be divided into before medical school, during medical school, during residency, or while in practice. An AMA survey of pregnancies during residencies in 1983 found that 2/3 of all women in practice had children. Almost half had had their first child during their residency or fellowship, and a quarter had had a second child during training.

In a study by Stewart and Robinson (1985) of 85 women psychiatrists, each participant was asked to comment on timing of pregnancy. There was general agreement that the first year of training was a poor choice. As the fourth year of residency is devoted to exam preparation, residents seemed to prefer the second and the third year of residency for childbearing. Graduates generally felt that waiting until training was completed was preferable.

Sinal et al (1988) did a large randomized study of over 900 women doctors. Participants had to be residency trained and under 50 years old. Sixty-four percent of the respondents had children, averaging 1.4 per respondent. Their first pregnancies occurred as follows: prior to medical school, 4%; during medical school, 7%; during internship, 11%; in another residency year, 32%; in fellowship, 13%; in practice 28%; and other, 5%. When asked about advice on pregnancy timing, nearly 70% suggested that the best time for a first pregnancy was after completion of the residency program.

Unplanned Pregnancies

Even the most knowledgable women (such as women physicians) have unplanned pregnancies, partly as a result of birth control failures. Several studies in the last five years have actually identified planned versus unplanned pregnancies in women physicians. Sayres et al (1986) found in her survey of 56 pregnancies that 77% were planned. Harris et al (1989, unpublished personal communication) found in her survey of over 200 pregnancies during residencies of both male and female residents, that 35% of all pregnancies during residency were unplanned. Nineteen percent of the unplanned conceptions occurred without the benefit of birth control. Sinal et al (1988), in a large randomized survey of over 900 women physicians, found that 77% of these womens' first pregnancies were planned.

Pregnancy Complications and Outcomes

Osborn et al (1988) surveyed 92 residents and 144 spouses of residents for pregnancy outcome. They identified among their white resident pregancies an increased risk of premature labor. No significant differences were found in prematurity, spontaneous and therapeutic abortions, or congenital anomalies between the two groups. Method of delivery and type of anesthetic used were also similar between the groups.

In the largest study done on women physicians, Phelan (1988) analyzed the responses from 1,197 women physicians. She found that the actual rate of medical and obstetrical complications is no different from that in the general population, except for the incidence of pregnany-induced hypertension (12%), as compared to the general population (5%). Phelan felt that this finding might represent an older maternal age rather than a true occupational hazard. In this study, the rate for spontaneous abortions was only 4%. Previous studies by Vaisman (1967) had reported an increased risk of spontaneous abortions among women exposed to exhaled anesthetic gases. However, a later study done by Pharoh et al (1977) could not identify an increased risk of spontaneous abortions among women anesthesiologists. Greenbaum et al (1987) studied the pregnancies of 454 obstetricians. Primigravida women who delivered during their residency training had statistically significant higher percentages of low birthweight infants. Seven and one-half percent of these infants showed intrauterine growth retardation.

At Mount Sinai School of Medicine, Butwell and Borgen (1986) found that among 94 residents pregnant at their institution, one quarter of them were absent from work at some time during their pregnancy. The majority of absences occurred during the third trimester as a consequence of a major medical complication. Other interesting findings in their study were that 21% of the women reported that their intention to have children affected their specialty choice. Almost 1/3 of the women who chose never to have children cited the incompatibility of their career with pregancy or childrearing as a major influencing factor.

Childbearing before Medical School

Pros

Psychologists Panmore, Daniels and Winegarten (Stephen) from the Westlake College Center for Research on Women studied 86 couples and concluded the following were advantages of having children when a woman was in her 20s:

1. *More Energy.* During this period of time, women are young and have a great deal of energy and enthusiasm to spend on childrearing.
2. *Fewer Non-child Responsibilities.* If the woman is not attending college during this time, there are relatively few other infringements on her time, allowing more time for child-rearing.
3. *Greater Flexibility.* When a woman is in her early 20s, she is not as set in her ways as when she grows older. This flexibility and less rigid personality structuree allows her to adjust to childrearing more readily.
4. *Less Infringement on Professional Growth.* Having children before medical school means that pregnancy and childbirth will not interfere with medical school or professional career.
5. *Less Financial Impact of Time Out.* After a woman starts to earn money, the family tends to become more dependent on the steady source of dollars. If the woman has not as yet begun to earn a good income, then the financial impact may be less.

Also:

6. *Physiologic Maximization.* The 20s are the best physiologic time for having children.

7. *Greater Maturity in Medical School.* Entering medical school later than the average student provides for greater maturity and a greater sense of the important aspects of the educational process.

Cons
1. *Greater Isolation in Medical School.* An older married student in medical school may have less peer support and be more isolated (Bluestone).
2. *Greater Responsibilities.* Childcare presents an additional major responsibility to those inherent in attending medical school.
3. *Lack of Role Models.* There tend to be few role models for the older female medical student with children.
4. *Resentment by Children.* Children may resent the mother's new time commitments and interests. This will, of course, vary from child to child, but a general rule would be that any major interest of this magnitude will draw resentment from children.
5. *Forced Redirection Upon Entry to Medical School.* The shift from childrearing to full-time study in medical school can be difficult. There will have to be a reorganization of priorities from childcare to schoolwork in order to maintain good academic standing. The previous independence that had often been enjoyed by the student may create trouble in coping with the ridigity and inflexibility experienced in medical training.

During Medical School

Most medical students believe that they will have their first child in ther 20s (Kaplan).

Pros
Many of the pros of having a child before medical school apply during medical school.
1. *More Energy.*
2. *Greater Flexibility.*
3. *Physiologic Maximization.*
4. *Less Financial Impact of Time Out.*

Cons
1. *Losing Academic Time.* Medical schools can be extremely rigid, though there are exceptions, and pregnancy with delivery during a school year may result in falling behind academically. There have

been medical students who took absolutely no time off, while others were forced to repeat an entire academic year (Kaplan).

2. *Lack of Role Models.* Not many others choose this route, making it difficult for individuals to see and follow patterns set by role models.

3. *Discouragement.* There is often little encouragement, and often active discouragement, of medical students wishing to have children (Pfeiffer).

4. *Multiple Responsibilities.*

5. *Forced Redirection.* The forced redirection in this case would be from full-time student to full-time student and mother.

6. *Inhibition of Identity Development.* During her early training, the woman student is developing her own feminine identity while simultaneously trying to develop the identity of a physician (Ordway). The establishment of the ego and sexual identities in a woman this age may be postponed if she is overwhelmed by the combined tasks of motherhood and completing medical school (Pfeiffer). The personality changes that will occur during medical school may result in the desire of different roles than those originally expected when the student was younger.

7. *Financial Burdens.* Unless there is a spouse with a high income or parents willing to support the efforts of the new family, the cost of medical school and childcare during medical school may be prohibitive (Bluestone).

8. *Peer Resentment.* Peers may resent the student-mother's outside responsibilities or her need to change schedules (Potter).

Childbearing during Residency

Pros

1. *Possibility of More Flexible Schedules.* There are flexible time-scheduled residencies available. Though no longer mandated, there are still a fair number of them available.

2. *Identity Development Completed.* Development of identity as a woman and as a physician will have occurred prior to residency (Pfeiffer, Ordway), and the woman will have made specific commitments to the profession.

3. *Physiologic Maximixation.* If the woman is still in her 20s, physiology is on her side (Bluestone).

4. *Reasonable Energy Levels.* Although a resident's energy level may be less than in her 20s, it will still be higher than in later years

(Bluestone, Baucom-Copeland). However, residency time commitments can interfere with this energy.

5. *Contribution to Physician Education.* The training program that does provide for childbearing among its female residents creates an excellent example of caring for the patient as a total human being (Heins 1977). It also allows direct observation of both the nurturing process and difficulties that today's women encounter in our society.

Cons

1. *Prolongation of Residency and Resulting Delay in Board-Certification.* Analysis of a survey performed by the American Academy of Family Physicians showed that of the 40% of the family practice residencies that had an existing maternity leave policy, almost 80% stated that an extension of the residency program was required as a result of that leave (Brunton). Similar delays in other specialty residencies may mean delay in board-certification for many specialties (Potter).

2. *Peer Resentment.* There is often resentment expressed by other residents if a pregnant resident or resident mother is given special considerations. In many instances, the pregnant resident has to make up call by having a heavier call schedule before or after delivery (Brunton): adjustment may be needed to allow the resident to be on more difficult rotations early in the pregnancy and less difficult rotations late in the pregnancy. This may create conflicts with peers (Baucom-Copeland). The female resident will encounter resistance and hostility if she calls attention to her different role and needs as a wife and mother.

3. *Physiologic Stress.* Residencies tend to be a time of physiologic stress related to loss of sleep and heavy work schedules (Potter). It can be difficult to sustain the stress of a pregnancy physiologically at the same time as experiencing the stress of late nights, missed sleep and meals. One also must wonder about the impact of such stresses on the unborn child (Kaplan).

4. *Mental Stress.* Sleep-deprived interns feel increased sadness and decreased vigor and social affection (Freidman). Numerous psychopathologic symptoms can develop and interns judge themselves to have abnormalities in cognitive perceptual and physiological areas of function (Freidman). To also have the mental attention to focus on a child can be difficult.

5. *Difficulty Finding Childcare Arrangements.* Because of the erratic and extended schedules of residents, it can be difficult to find

appropriate and financially feasible childcare arrangements. If the spouse is also a physician or resident, problems can be compounded by overlapping night call schedules.

6. *Difficulties with Breast-Feeding.* The more erratic the schedule and the less time taken off after delivery, the more difficult it can be to breast-feed an infant. Although breast-feeding problems may occur at any time, residency is the time period in a woman physician's life that they tend to be the worst.

7. *Discouragement.* Just as during medical school, many residencies actively discourage residents from having children.

Childbearing During Practice

Pros

1. *Control.* Control is the biggest advantage of having a child during the practice years. A woman has very little control over her schedule during the training years. However, once out of the residency, she can choose her practice situation, and has the option of choosing a practice with flexibility in scheduling.

2. *Affordability.* Once earning more money, it is easier to afford children. Childcare options are greater when there is money to support them.

3. *Matured Personality.* The personality of the woman physician will have matured more completely and the role of physician will be better established. The woman is more certain of herself as a human being and potential mother (Bluestone).

4. *Stable Spouse Relationship.* The relationship with a husband is usually more stable and established with additional years of marriage, providing a more secure base for children.

Cons

1. *Fertility limitations.* Those who delay childbirth in order to complete training obviously feel the pressure of the biological time clock. The number of children one can conceive in a given period of time is limited. Fertility peaks in the early 20s and is on a decline in the 30s, though it does not decline significantly until the late 30s or early 40s (Bluestone).

2. *Congenital Anomalies.* After 30, the chances of abnormalities in children begin to rise and increase with every passing year. Down's Syndrome occurs in one out of 885 births at the age of 30, once in 365 births at 35, and once in 287 births at 36 (Bluestone). By

the time a mother is 39, the chances of having a Down's child is one in 176.

3. *Maternal and Fetal Morbidity and Mortality.* Older women face a somewhat greater chance of death from childbirth than younger mothers. According to the Centers for Disease Control, there are seven maternal deaths for every 100,000 women ages 20 to 24, as compared to 44 deaths for every 100,000 women in women over the age of 35. Women pregnant for the first time over age 35 have an especially high rate of perinatal death (Bluestone).

4. *Less Time for Career.* Having children generally means less time for the career. In practice, this may mean less money and perhaps less prestige. In academic medicine, it may mean slower (or no) promotion.

This summary of the pros and cons of the various times to have children underestimates at least two important factors. One concerns fears inherent in delaying childbirth and the other concerns the emotional impact of having children.

Career women such as female physicians often delay having children until they are more established in their careers, such as during or after residency. Fertility decreases as a woman gets older. For this reason, women physicians typically fear the impact of waiting on their childbearing ability. What happens if she significantly delays childbearing then cannot get pregnant? Will she or her spouse be able to accept this, or will the guilt of believing that she might have been able to get pregnant if she had only tried earlier, be overwhelming? Is she tempting fate, risking losing the experience of having children, by waiting? Whether or not this is physiologically true, the fear is real and may well be a reason that many women physicians do not delay even longer.

One should also consider the emotional impact of childbirth when deciding at what stage in one's career to have children. Women may have unanticipated feelings of contentment upon birth of a child (Ordway). The child may stimulate a stronger sense of attachment and pleasure than the mother had expected. Children can be very enticing and fun, but the professional woman may think this will not apply to her to the same extent as to the general public. When the child arrives, and the woman does experience a great amount of contentment and pleasure with the child, the career suddenly may diminish in importance. One hears of women who have children and then quit work, even when they had not origianlly planned to do so. The female physician often thinks this will not happen to her. When the child arrives, and she has stronger bonding and attachment than expected, she must deal with how to prioritize the child and her career. Should this happen during a time that she feels little or no option in terms of her work situation, she may have even more guilt than may accompany childibrth at a time when it would be easier to have more time with the child. Women should realize the possibility of unanticipated contentment and consider it in planning.

Maternity Leave

Leaving a newborn child is an extremely individual matter and each woman may not be able to identify her own personal needs until after the child is born. Physiologically, many women can return to work fairly quickly after having a child, although a very heavy schedule may be hard to maintain, and those who have C-Sections may require additional time to recuperate. Emotionally, though, the best time to return to work is quite variable. Because of the uniqueness of the needs involved, each physician will have to determine her own leave time.

The Federal Pregnancy Discrimination Act of 1978 forbids an employer from discriminating against pregnant employees. The law does not state that a certain amount of maternity leave must be granted, but it does state that if a sick leave exists, that maternity leave must be equal. Most other industrialized nations provide a minimum of 12 weeks of leave (Sayres). England allows 18 weeks and France 16 weeks.

The time taken for childbearing is a highly individualized issue. There are abundant stories in female medical circles of women delivering over Thanksgiving vacation and being back in class or at work the following Monday. Luckily this superwoman compelx is uncommon.   In the Indianapolis group mentioned in Chapter 10 on child care, the shortest time taken for maternity leave was ten days. One obstetrician returned to work at that time to perform a C-Section on one of her patients. Several other women in this group said that they also resumed part-time work in ten days. For those taking little time off, the most frequently cited reason was that the woman was unable to tolerate being home any longer. However, another female obstetrician stated that, at 13 weeks, she returned to work and continued to have crying spells for days after leaving the child. The average time off appeared to be somewhere between four and six weeks.

Sayres (1986) found that most institutions were unprepared for maternity leave. Four-fifths of the residency programs surveyed had no written maternity leave policy. No resident quit a program because of pregancy in her study. Sixty three percent of the women took no time off before their delivery. Leave after the birth of the baby averaged eight weeks. Many of the residents in her study worked double duty before delivery in anticipation of maternity related leave. Nine percent had worked out a part-time residency schedule post partum.

In Sinal's (1988) study, only 33% of the respondents reported that their training or work sites had maternity leave policies at the time of their first pregnancy. Sixty percent took leaves of six weeks or less. Twenty-one percent took seven weeks to three months. These findings were very similar to the previous findings of the 1984 AMA study and Sayre's Study at Harvard. In Canada, where national policy allows 15 weeks paid benefits and two weeks unpaid for maternity leave, the average time taken off by residents is 16 weeks (Stewart and Robinson).

The best and most creative maternity leave policy will do a resident little good if she is rendered ineligible to sit for her boards because of it. Of the 22 speciality boards, 14 have no specific policy, or leave the policy up to the directors (Bernstein 1988). The American Board of Pediatrics allows only three months of absence during the three years of training. On the other extreme, the American Board of Allergy and Immunology has no attendance requirement for candidates (Wynn). Restrictive time require- ments may discourage a woman from taking her boards if she must sit for them at a later date.

Summary

Life is full of choices and few are larger than deciding whether and when to have children. This is compounded for someone pursuing a profession, particularly one that has many demands and rewards similar to motherhood. Most female physicians do have children, and must consider physiologic, emotional and practical factors in deciding when to have the children. For those who do have children, the demands and frustrations, as well as rewards, can be great.

References

AMA Ad Hoc Committee on Women. Maternity leave for residents. Report to the Board of Trustees, American Medical Association, Chicago, Illinois,1984.

Baucom-Copeland et al. Pregnant resident: Career conflict? J Am Med Wom Assoc 1983;38(4):103-105.

Bernstein AE. Maternity leave for housestaff: Moving from advocacy to advice. J Am Med Wom Assoc 1988;43(3):85-88.

Bluestone N. Marriage and medicine. J Am Med Wom Assoc 1965;20(11): 1048-1053.

Brunton SM, Ostergaard D. Report on a workshop on maternity and patenity leave held at the directors of family practice residency programs workshop, 1982.

Butwell NB, Borgen RE. Pregnancy during residency. Letter to the Editor. N Engl J Med 1986;314(25):1646.

Dykman R, Stalnaker J. Survey of women physicians graduating from medical school 1925-1940. J Med Educ 1957;32:3-38.

Freidman R, Bigger T, Kornfeld D. The intern and sleep loss. N Engl J Med 1971;285(4):201-203.

Greenbaum A, Minkoff H, Blade D. Pregnancy among obstetricians: A comparison of births before, during and after residency. Am J Obstet Gynecol 1987;157: 79-84.

Heins M. Medicine and motherhood. JAMA 1982;249(2):209-210.

Heins M, Smack S, Martindale L, et al. Comparison of productivity of women and men physicians. JAMA 1977;237(23):2514-2517.

Kaplan H. Women physicians--The more effective recruitment and utilization of their talents and their resistance to it. The Woman Physician 1970;25(9):561-570.

Medica Survey. Medica, Fall 1983, p. 4-5.

Ordway J. Professional women's unanticipated contented feelings after the birth of a child. J Am Med Wom Assoc 1980;35(10):240-245.

Osborn LM, Harris DL, Reading JC, Prather MB. Female residents not at increased risk for adverse pregnancy outcome. Research in Medical Education 1988 Proceedings of the 27th Annual Conference, Association of American Medical Colleges, Chicago, November, 1988.

Pfeiffer RJ. Early adult development in the medical student. Mayo Clin Proc 1983;58:127-134.

Pharoh P, Alberman E, Chamberlain G. Outcome of pregnancy among women in anesthetic practice. Lancet 1977;1:34-36.

Phelan ST. Pregnancy during residency: II. Obstetric complications. Obstet Gynecol 1988;72(3):431-436.

Potter RL. Resident, woman, wife, mother: Issues for women in training. J Am Med Wom Assoc 1983;38(4):103-105.

Sayres M, Wyshak G, Denterlein G. Pregnancy during residency. N Engl J Med 1986;314(7):418-423.

Sinal S, Weavil P, Camp MG. Survey of women physicians on issues relating to pregancy during a medical career. J Med Educ 1988;63:531-538.

Stephen B. What's the best time to have a baby? Redbook, February 1983, p. 36.

Stewart DE, Robinson GE. Combining motherhood with psychiatric training and practice. Can J Psychiatry 1985;30:28-34.

Vaisman A. Working conditions in surgery and their effects on the health of anesthesiologists. Eksp Khir Anesteziol 1967;3:44-49.

Wynn SR. Pregnancy during residency. Letter to the Editor. N Engl J Med 1986; 314(25):1646.

"I am a person whose values from the 1960s have not waned, rather they have deepened. My commitment to the social change has taken the form of a long term dedication to the teaching and practicing of family medicine in an inner city health center, where awareness of our society's inequalities is ever-present. I like to think that I practice in an egalitarian fashion; I attempt to put patients in charge of interactions as much as possible. By this I don't mean that I hold them responsible for their health (or sickness), rather that I try to let the time be their time with me, to use the way they think necessary. This means I am committed to understanding and working through patient agendas, not just doctor-based agendas.

Feminism is a strong current in my orientation. In my practice, feminism means struggling to enable women to discover their strengths, and to recover from the innumerable restrictions, hurts, and violations that have curtailed their freedom to grow and choose for themselves and their children. Physical and sexual abuse are frequent realities in the current and past lives of my patients. I believe that helping them heal from these assaults is one of the most rewarding tasks of feminist practice.

Nonetheless to say, this is not short work. I have made my *practice* and not my career the centerpiece of my work. This means that I have chosen to remain in one setting for the past fifteen years, the same site where I completed by family practice residency. A doctor used to be a person who came and stayed. Staying means staying in labor, staying in the practice, and staying in the community. I believe that the real work of family practice cannot be done in a few years, that the magic in the work lies in all the shared history.

Rare is the woman who has the good fortune to find a life partner who shares equally in her values and her commitment to her work. When Richard Schmitt, a committed socialist and feminist philosopher, joined me in Worcester in 1983, I knew that I was such a woman. Our daily joint engagement in both intellectual and family work make my life rich and full. The depth of our relationship has enabled each of us to confront painful past histories and turn our understandings into growth in our work.

I am employed part-time. What this means is that I am in the health center a little more than two and a half days; I take one night per week of call and eight weekends a year. I do obstetrics and attempt to deliver my own patients when I am not on call. For this I am paid at 67% of a full-time salary, which is ample to live on. The two days I am at home, I spend reading and writing. This arrangement enables me to pursue my ideas as freely as possible with only occasional clinical interruptions, which are, after all, what I read and write about anyway.

We have two children, Addie, 6, in first grade, and Eli, 16 months, at family day care; three acres on a pond; a large garden; and a sister city project with a town in Nicaragua. How is it possible to do it all? First, for many years even before I met him, Richard had also chosen to work for pay on a half-time basis. His career was well established, and his position secure. In practice, he teaches first semester and has nine months to read and write. Secondly, we share all the responsibilities around the children equally, including transportation and doctors' appointments. Third, I spend no time commuting; our home is ten minutes from the health center and the hospitals. Fourth, we have forty hours a week of child care; Addie joins Eli at Debra Keating's family day care home after school for snacks and play until five o'clock. The days we are home are really available to us. Lastly, we watch no television and do not have a VCR. Our children's time with us, and ours with them, is intense, busy, engaged.

For me, my various roles--doctor, teacher, writer, mother, lover--are compatible not conflicting. In many ways, each role is essential to the well-being of the others. Take away any, and all would suffer.

A sharing life partner, part-time employment, truly open time for creative work, excellent day care--these things are the essential ingredients in my recipe. And these are exactly what any person with children needs in stretching to reach his or her full potential. That's why I will keep working towards a society based on equal relationships, meaningful work for adequate pay, and respect for the enormity of human possibility. In the meantime, I will continue to struggle against oppressive and hierarchical relationships in families, between races, and between countries. I am centered in the deep connections which link my politics, my personal life, and my practice.

Lucy M. Candib, M.D.
Family Practice, Neighborhood Health Center
early 40s, Permanently Co-habitating
with Richard Schmitt and Two Children

12
Child-Rearing

Even today, as society changes its attitudes toward who can provide child care, the husband of a woman physician who assumes responsibility for child care is still a rarity (Rapoport). The intent to share family responsibilities is frequently made before pregnancy, but once a child is born, child care is the responsibility of the woman (Nadelson 1979). One of the major concerns of young women physicians is how to integrate their marriage, their families, and their careers (Konanc). Most medical students anticipate having children, but foresee childbearing as interfering with their performance in medical school, residency, and later in private practice (Konanc).

There are no easy solutions to combining a career and family life, but the woman physician should know her options. This chapter will explore the options are available for child care, how women physicians are currently handling child care, and the cost both monetarily and personally for surrogate care of the children. Hopefully, understanding the problems, and recognizing the limitations, options and needs, will reduce the stresses involved with the dual roles of mother and physician.

National Figures

In 1986, 4.8 million mothers with children under 3 were in the workforce (Bernstein). This represents almost exactly 50% of all mothers with children of this age. By the year 2000, it is expected that 75% of the mothers of the very young will enter the workforce. Currently the majority of children are in care that is under the supervision of a relative; 25.7% are cared for in their own homes; 43.8% are cared for in other homes, and 18.8% are in daycare centers. The rest are unknown. Almost 95% of the daycare is informal and unregulated. About 70% of working mothers used more than one type of child care arrangement (Kamerman).

A Gallup Poll released in September 1983 showed that one out of four dual parent households with children had a working mother as primary breadwinner with a father who was staying home and taking care of the children (National Survey). This is much different than in the world of medicine where it is uncommon for husbands of female physicians to do so (Rapoport). 85% of the men physicians reported that their wives took complete care of their children (Rapoport).

One of the useful innovations in child care (Kamerman) is the Information and Referral (I & R) services, created to improve coordination of children and child care providers. I & Rs also work to educate parents about the characteristics of a high quality child care service while leaving the parent the ultimate decision of which service to choose. California provides a public subsidy for I & R services. A few progressive employers have also established such services for their employees as a low cost alternative to the direct sponsorship of a child care program.

There are a number of different for-profit services that locate child care for parents, particularly in metropolitan areas. They frequently charge a set fee for providing a certain number of interviews. Although the service can be expensive, it may be worth the money if good child care results.

Current Child Care Used by Woman Physicians and Its Cost

Child care is perhaps the biggest bane of the woman physician mother's existence. Stewart and Robinson (1985) found in their Canadian study that 84% of psychiatrist mothers reported numerous concerns over child care. Virtually all mentioned the need for emergency back up coverage. The majority of studies done on child care for woman physicians were done in the 60s and 70s. During that time, daycare was a very unpopular method of child care. In one study, one-third of all women physicians were opposed to day-care centers for their children (Heins 1977). Things have apparently changed somewhat. In a 1983 Medica survey (Medica), 18% of women physicians relied on live-in help; 29% on daily help coming to their homes; 20% on daycare and 20% on other child care outside the home. About 19% of the younger age group had family members providing care. When women physicians were asked to name the most successful types of child care (Sinal 1989), they listed daily caretaker in the home or live-in caretaker most frequently.

Few hospitals cater to the needs of their physicians in training or to their nursing staff. According to a study by the Association of American Medical Colleges in 1987 (Rippis), only 60 of the responding 373 teaching hospitals reported on-site daycare for the children of housestaff. The charges for the service ranged from $45 to $100 dollars a week. Even these hospitals did not take into account call schedules, and only five stayed open until midnight (Rippis 1989).

The "Child Care Tax Credit" became a significant benefit in 1976 and was increased as part of the 1981 Economic Recovery Tax Act (Kamerman). If parents earn enough to pay taxes, but earn under $10,000, they can take a tax credit of up to $720 on expenses of $2,400 for one child and $1,440 on expenses of $4,800 for two or more. If the parents income is above $28,000, the credit is a maximum of $480 for one child and $960 for two or more. This would appear of minimal help to women physicians. Although a woman physician cannot be productive without the support of child care services, the true cost of such services is not tax deductible (Heins 1979).

Choosing Child Care Services

The people that a woman physician hires to provide child care and household help are critical to her. The effort and care taken to select a reliable, warm and honest person will be invaluable in the end. It is wise to choose a person who uses child-rearing techniques and has standards similar to the parents' own. If this person is also expected to do household chores, the standards of cleanliness must be similar. This will ease the physician's worries about her family and provide her the physicial and mental freedom to pursue her career (Scher).

There is no guarantee of quality in child care services. Federal standards for child care services were eliminated when Congress passed the Reagan Administration's social services block grant legislation. It is now up to the states to set standards and to enforce them. Some states have inadequate standards and, even in states with standards, they may be applicable to only a portion of child care programs. Some states do not enforce the standards they do have, whereas other states are quite diligent about enforcement. It is hoped that the quality of child care will improve as the competition increases among providers (Kamerman).

Plenty of time is needed to find child care. A minimum of four to six weeks is suggested. If this length of time coincides with the time taken off for maternity leave, the decision may be made to wait until the child is born to hunt for child care. Some women are uncomfortable with not having arrangements made before the child is born, though, and will choose to select child care as early as possible. However, many child care workers or centers will not take reservations months in advance. If a person is being hired to come into the home, an additional two weeks should be added, because this process takes longer.

It may also take time to decide on the type of child care that is desired. There are advantages and disadvantages to each. The following paragraphs discuss each type in ascending order of cost.

Daycare centers seem to be an unpopular choice for child care for women physicians. However, they are the lowest cost alternative, and this monetary feature can be attractive. The major advantages are:

1. They are generally the least costly alternative.
2. They are readily available.
3. They frequently have educational programs for the children.
4. Children have the opportunity to socially interact with other children their own age.
5. They are frequently regulated by state or local laws.
6. There is less reliance on a single caretaker.

Major disadvantages to daycare centers are:

1. They have set hours of operation, which often do not coincide with the work hours of physicians.
2. Many will not accept infants.
3. There are large numbers of children with relatively few caretakers. As a result, there is less individual attention for each child.
4. The large number of children leads to the spread of infection.
5. They are inflexible in their arrangements.
6. Very few will care for ill children.
7. The mother may be asked to participate in administrative activities.

Child care in someone else's home is the next least expensive choice. How well this works for an individual will depend on the person taking care of the child. The situation may or may not be regulated, depending on the locale and the number of children cared for by the individual. These arrangements tend to be more flexible than daycare centers, have fewer children, and can provide more individual attention. Some will care for children who are ill, or keep children all night when the physician is on-call. If the caretaker becomes ill or something else prevents the caretaker from caring for the children, the parents must find alternative arrangements. Costs for this type of care averaged $220 per year in North Carolina in 1988 (Kebschull).

Child care in one's own home means the child does not have to be 'put-together' every morning for transport elsewhere--a major advantage. However, one is dependent on the promptness and reliability of the caretaking individual, and back-up arrangements must be readily available. The child care worker may care for an ill child. The privacy and security of household possessions should be considered, since household workers have been known to discuss private matters and to steal. These arrangements may have flexible hours, and flexible requirements. Some can transport children to pre-school, school or sport activities. Some will also do household work, which can be a great boon. Having someone else in the home all day, as well as having the child(ren) home all day can mean that there is more cleaning to be done. This arrangement is basically unregulated, except for the rules that apply to employment.

If an employee who works in a home is paid $50 or more in a three-month period, it is necessary to file annual W-2 forms (statement of income, tax withheld and social security taxes) and form 942 with the IRS (to pay employee's social security taxes). One must pay at least the current minimum wage ($3.35 per hour, minimum $135 for a 40-hour week, figures which are scheduled to change). Social security taxes are equal to 15.02% of income, which either the employer and employee can pay 50% or the employer can elect to pay all of it. With a single employee, the employer can either withhold Federal income taxes or agree with the employee that the employee will file quarterly income tax statements. For these things, the physician needs both Federal and state employer identification numbers. Unemployment taxes must also be paid to Federal and state governments.   Worker's compensation insurance is usually available through local insurance agencies. Taking care of these multiple items is time-consuming, expensive (amounting to about 25% over the salary paid), and frustrating (because of the necessity of dealing with Federal and state bureaucracies). In addition, the rules are subject to change. Alternatively, live-in help can be hired through agencies who will take care of such items but charge to do so. Young women from abroad or other immigrants are sometimes hired to work in the home, at which time knowledge of immigration laws and visas is important.

Live-in help is the most expensive, but has several advantages. Live-in workers will usually also do housework and care for an ill child. There is greatest flexibility in terms of the hours of child care, although even live-ins need vacation and time off. There must be space available in the home for a private room(s) for the individual, and there is significantly less privacy for the family. The security of household possessions must again be considered.

Cost The cost of child care ranged widely depending on the type of care provided and the region of the country. In Florida and New York in 1983, a daycare center for a preschooler cost about $45 a week and for an infant or a toddler about $55 a week (Kamerman). By contrast, in New Jersey and Philadelphia, the cost was about $75 a week for a preschooler and $96 for a toddler, while infant care was as high as $126 a week. Obviously, without financial help from a spouse or family much of what is available is beyond the price range of a woman physician who is still in training.

(Kamerman). Overall, women physicians (Medica Survey) averaged $91 a week for child care: outside child care averaged about $76 a week; if the child was cared for in the home, the cost averaged $115 a week. Rippis (1989) found the charge for hospital-provided daycare was $45 to $100 a week.

Using Family Members for Child Care

There is very little written about using family members for child care; however, it would appear to be a viable alternative. Family members may be willing to go the extra mile and be flexible in terms of hours. On the other hand, there is an apparent loss of control, as the employer-employee relationship may be constrained when family members have different ideas of childrearing.

Finding and Choosing a Day Care Center

The requirements for selecting a daycare center are similar from state to state, but choosing a daycare center can be a complicated task. With some guidance, a concerned parent can successfully evaluate the quality of a daycare program. Several lay texts provide a blueprint for evaluation of centers, and books such as "Quality Daycare" by Richard Endsley (1981) is a good general guide. The American Academy of Pediatrics has also published a book entitled "Health in Daycare: A Manual for Health Professionals" (Deitch). The chapters in the book describe the child care setting, the interplay of child and professionals; and the health, growth, and developmental factors that may require a physician's attention. The book was meant to serve as a reference for the topics it covers and is highly recommended.

It is a good idea for parents to drop in unexpectedly on whatever option is chosen. This provides an opportunity to see the routine supervision of the children. It is also a good opportunity to check the general cleanliness, type and quality of the food, and any other areas of concern.

Care In Another Home

If the physician's home is located in an areas where there are a lot of young families with children, it may be possible to find daycare in the home of a neighbor or someone in the immediate area. Many of these arrangements are found through the grapevine and the informal networks that exist in neighborhood and work situations. In many states, homes do not need to be licensed unless they offer daycare to more than five children, including the children of the daycare provider. If the woman is doing this professionally, she may take the option of being licensed to protect the children she cares for, the parents, and herself. It is possible to ask that the provider also be bonded. For specific information contact the State Board of Health in the respective state. Some child care workers request that the income not be reported for Federal income tax or social security purposes; the employing physician must be aware that this is illegal. To claim a tax credit for the child care expenses, the physician must provide the name of the child care provider to the Internal Revenue Service.

Care After School

Once the child enters the school system, arrangements for child care change. They must now encompass the new problem of transportation to and from school plus care before and after school hours. If the physician has the luxury of a live-in or come-in housekeeper, this should be included in her job description and special attention paid to her car availability.

For those who are not so fortunate, special arrangements must be made for transportation. If the school bus transports children to and from your neighborhood, use it. But alternative arrangements still must be made for missed buses or outside activities lasting beyond regular school hours. If the physician relies heavily on a neighbor or other individual for transportation of her children, she should consider payment or some reciprocal service for the time and effort.

Some schools and child care centers offer after-school arrangements. Some child care centers send buses to schools to transport children to the daycare center. Similar arrangements can be made with a trusted neighbor, family member, or paid employee. Neighborhood teens might be interested in the job, but may be less reliable because of their own after school activities.

While there are many 'latchkey' children in the United States, i.e., those who go home to an empty house and stay there alone until the parent arrives home from work, it is not an option chosen by many women physicians. This arrangement works best for mature and responsible children who have activities outlined for them and ready telephone access to their parent. Early work on latchkey children found them to be more fearful and lonely, but four studies done since 1982 have found no differences between latchkey children and children cared for by an adult in a home (Zylke, Dec 16, 1988). However, being removed from adult supervision may make an adolescent more susceptible to peer pressure (Zylke, Dec 16, 1988).

Child Care During the Summer

What to do with school-age children home for the summer can be a perplexing problem. Some of the larger daycare centers offer summer programs including day camps, frequent field trips, swimming lessons and structured outside games. YMCAs and YWCAs also provide many activities. The local recreation department can often be of assistance. Some churches offer special programs as well. Unfortunately, summer programs are not as prevalent as most working women would like and the ideal program may not be available in a location convenient for transportation.

Another method of summer child care is to hire a responsible teenager to babysit for the summer. Usually there is an industrious teen who is suitable. Summer camps should also be considered.

Guidelines for Hiring a Care Provider For in the Home

These guidelines apply to both live-ins as well as other caretakers who will be coming into the home. In this situation, the woman physician will be essentially acting as her own personnel service. The method used for hiring caretakers in the home should not be different from that used for hiring office personnel. One should take the same care and planning as for other employer-employee relationships.

The first step is to prepare a list of qualifications needed. Next, develop the application form. If the application form from the office practice is suitable, it can be used; it not, one needs to be created. After this, a notice can be posted in the city paper, the neighborhood paper, or in churches. The listing should include the job available and the minimum requirements. Word of mouth from employees, patients, other medical personnel or even fellow church members also appear to be important sources of child care information. Ask all applicants to mail a resume. In small towns, this method does not appear to be as effective as in metropolitan areas.

When posting a notice, it may be wiser to use a post office box number than to give out a home phone number or address. With public posting, there may be an abundance of initial replies, up to 100-200 in a large metropolitan area. Estimates are that perhaps half of these will meet the minimum requirements listed in the notice.

After receiving the initial replies, the respondents should be pre-screened. Final application forms should only be sent to those who may be viable for the job. Again a post office box may be best. For ten to fifteen of the applicants, all references should be called or asked to provide written letters of reference. This is a must!! Telephone calls may yield more negative information pertinent to the hiring. Estimates are that half of the references will be bogus, and calling references will save interviewing time and possibly prevent hiring the wrong child care worker. It is often wise to ask directly about possible alcohol and drug use of the proposed worker. Interviewing can be done at home, but the formal setting of the physician office may be preferred. Questions to be asked in the interview should be predetermined and should include all vital aspects of child care. These may include punishment, stimulation, dietary habits, smoking, alcohol and drug use, illnesses, use of car seats, vacations, and ownership of a car.

A written job description also helps to solidify actual job expectations. The job description (see sample) should be individualized for what is believed to be needed from the caretaker. The range of jobs may be from simple babysitting responsibilities to all grocery shopping and buying of clothing for the children to a variety of household chores. Discussing the job description with the applicant can prevent a lot of trouble later.

The next topic to discuss is cost. It is wise to ask the applicant exactly how much she feels the particular job is worth. How much money is spent will be dependent on their expectations and on the usual rates in the local area. One must pay at least the current minimum wage. The authors have found that in 1989, the costs for in-home child care ranges from a low of $150 dollars a week with one child, to as high as $450 for 3 children in an East coast town.

As with any employee, the possibility that one day the caretaker will need to be fired must be considered. A probationary period where there is a review of the performance on a regular basis should be a part of the job. During the prearranged performance review, the difficulties that either party is having can be discussed. The caretaker should be fired if not meeting expectations. It is more difficult to deal with inadequate child care and irresponsibility on a day-to-day basis than it is to fire a person.

The Effect of Surrogate Care on Children

The American tradition of the mother staying at home raising the child provokes feelings of guilt and inadequacy in every women physician as she leaves her child in the morning. It is, however, a distinctly American tradition. Years ago, other countries developed daycare centers and domestic helpers more extensively, making leisure and social acitvities possible for all mothers (Women..Med World News). In the USA the employed wife enjoys substantially less leisure time and sleep than her husband (Battle 1985).

Up until a few years ago daycare was felt to be a "woman's issue," and not taken very seriously. The issues surrounding the crisis on the child care front were finally realized and became a major issue in the 1988 presidential campaign. (Zylke, December 9, 1988)

Female physicians themselves are not taught the current literature on the mother and infant attachment or on maternal deprivation (Potter). Intuitively, it is felt that the mother and infant interaction in child-rearing is paramount. Freud produced guilt in mothers in the 1920s by espousing the belief that mothers were considered to be responsible for the emotional and psychological well-being of their children. This was reinforced by Dr. Spock in the 1950s when he wrote about the importance of the mother's presence in meeting a child's emotional needs (Scott). Medical organizational attitudes and policies have traditionally reflected the concept that the presence of the biological mother is necessary during the child's formative years (Baucum-Copeland). It now seems a rather formidable task, and probably unnecessary, to feel solely responsible for the psychological development of any person.

We do not have a lot of hard data regarding the physical and psychological status of the offspring of medical mothers (Bernstein). The optimal quantity or quality of time for mother-child interaction is not known, nor is whether or not an infant needs a single identified caretaker for most of her/his waking hours or not. Perhaps several caring adults can be as effective as one. The answers are not obvious (Avery). For the most part, it is felt that children can adapt to as many as three or four different caring people available on a regular basis (Winter). Studies show that infants are able to form multiple attachments, and, therefore, fathers and/or other caretakers can be important attachments in their early development (Potter). Extensive studies on infants do not exist because this type of care was not used much before women recently began entering the workforce in large numbers. There is some evidence that extensive nonparental care may cause an insecure attachement of some infants. The exact significance of these findings are still hotly debated (Zylke, December 9, 1988).

Scharff (1985) feels that the idea of quality time is a myth. A woman physician returning home after a long day at work is usually worn out. The mother then tries to reunite with a child who is also either tired or frantic or both. The time the two have together may be valuable to both of them, but it is not necessarily "quality." Perhaps, however, it is the societal definition of "quality" that is the myth. Many parents, including women staying in the home, do not spend much time directed at the children, in such activities as long reading sessions or playing goal-directed games.

Hoffman (1974) pointed out that the effects on children of their mothers working depended on a variety of factors, including the nature of the employment, the general family circumstances, social class, the age and sex of the children, and, in particular, child care arrangements. Hoffman goes on to state that the working mother provides a largely positive role model for her children. There is no solid evidence that the mother's employment status in and of itself leads to juvenile delinquency or other forms of social or psychological problems in school-age children (Hoffman). Howell (1985) feels that maternal employement affects the child only through the direct exposure to a female engaged in paid work. She feels that when high quality, stable surrogate care is provided, there is no evidence that the infants of employed mothers are harmed in any way. Nadelson and Notman (1981) state that separation itself may not be a major factor responsible for attachment failure; rather, the pressure and fatigue of maternal stresses are more influential than a lack of time between the mother and child. If a working woman projects positive feelings about her job and her sense of worth as a working mother, the children will respond to this. If she projects negative guilt, they will also pick up on these feelings as well (Potter).

In an article by Heins and Stillman (1983), the majority of pediatricians surveyed reported few differences between chidren of employed mothers and those whose mothers remained at home. There appeared to be an overrepresentation of female and younger pediatricians among the respondents, but the investigators believed them to be reasonably representative of practicing pediatricians. The pediatricians were asked to compare children of employed mothers in their practices with children of mothers who did not work outside the home. The majority of the respondents believed that there was no difference in child development, academic difficulties or emotional problems; however, nearly two-thirds reported that children of employed mothers developed more acute infections. Nearly half believed that children whose mothers were employed outside the home functioned more independently and that children developed stronger attachments to mothers who did not work outside the home. When asked how old the child should be before the mother goes to work (assuming the mother wants to work for her own fulfillment), 29% of the respondents said it did not matter; 17% said 3 months or less, 26% 3 years, 36% when the child started school, and 1% said never.

Studies of some middle and upper class women who worked in careers by choice showed that they tended to be overprotective and over solicitous of their younger children (Scher). This behavior decreased as the child reached adolescence. This may well be the result of the mother's guilt rather than the work itself. Other studies indicated that professional women tend to have greater self-esteem and a sense of competence than nonworking mothers which is reflected in how their own children viewed them (Scher).

It is in the teen years that Howell feels we see the most regular and clear cut benefits from an employed mother. She feels that children of employed mothers are likely to see adult capabilities that are not limited by sexual stereotypes. There is some tendency for adolescent children to rebel and want to be exactly opposite of their family. Some females state they will never work outside the house, and boys may claim they want a wife who stays home. In actuality as they enter adulthood they tend to follow in their parents' footsteps (Howell).

In a study by Rapaport and Rapaport (1971), children of dual-career couples showed independence and resourcefulness. By helping with the family, they contributed to the overall family function and became an equal sharer in the family rights. Children in these types of families showed pride in their parents' accomplishments, which tended to raise a child's level of competence and involvement in a wide range of interests of both of the parents. There is a greater range of role models for children of both sexes. Neurotic difficulties, confused identification and other psychiatric disturbances of the children of dual-career couples appeared to be a product of bad management of child care rather than the particular family structure in and of itself. Current research is aimed at trying to decipher the multiple factors that affect a child's well being. Many researchers feel that the most significant factor will turn out to be quality of care. Quality care is composed of many factors including a good staff-child ratio, small group size, adequate training of the caretaker, and stability of care (Zylke).

A child's willingness and ability to adapt to outside care is important. Physical and emotional well-being and pride in their mother's accomplishments make a child's acceptance of her curtailed activities in many other areas of his/her life easier. Conversely, a child's independence and sense of responsibility are all reinforcement for her. There also appears to be a direct correlation between a working mother and high achievement in children, although there is certainly no guarantee (Scher).

The Wellness of Our Children

As more and more children enter daycare situations, it is becoming more evident that there may be a high toll to pay in terms of the child's health. The strongest predictor for increased infections was the number of other children in the room. Children in daycare centers were 4.5 times more likely to be hospitalized than those in other settings (Bell). Diarrheal diseases have been a common problem in daycare centers, and recent studies have found outbreaks of more uncommon pathogens including giardiasis (Steketee).

It is of interest that, in general, physicians tend to take their children to the doctor at later stages in an illness than the general public (Wasserman). The children also tend to be referred to specialists directly by their parents. There is also less documentation of a psychosocial history in the chart of physician's child. In a study of adolescent children of physicians presenting for psychiatric help, no typical syndrome could be identified (Stein and Leventhal).

Dealing with Guilt

Women are socially conditioned to find gratification in more diverse ways than strictly from their professional success (Angel). As a result, in past years many women physicians have stayed at home with their young children, believing that the rewards of this outweighed the cost of their interrupting their medical careers (Kaplan). Today, more women physicians are choosing to work longer hours. The price paid for expansion in the medical field may be an overwhelming guilt about the associated lack of time during the early developmental stages of the children. Even knowing the current literature on child care does not remove that nagging sensation that is felt by every working mother deep in her heart--best known as guilt.

When deciding what type of child care is suitable, everyone in the extended family is apt to give conflicting advice. The couple must decide for themselves and must be confident that the best decision has been made. They are the ones who have to live with the decision every day.

Summary

Child care will continue to be one of the biggest problems that a woman physician has to address. The appropriate child care that is most suitable to the parents and the working situations should be chosen. Effective child care permits the woman physician the freedom to pursue her career more actively. Although the woman physician often feels guilty about surrogate child care, children have been shown to be capable of developing multiple attachments without harm. There seems to be a positive relationship between working mothers and high achievement of the children. New options for dealing with difficult child care issues may develop as more and more women enter the workforce.

SAMPLE JOB DESCRIPTION

Smith-Jones Family Helper

Job includes:

1. Child Care: Complete care of the baby in our absence. This is top priority. No other responsibility or personal need is to interfere with this.
2. Routine House Cleaning: Making beds, change sheets every week. Dust furniture, scrub and wax floors, vacuum carpets, clean bathrooms and wash dishes.
   a. Clean stove, refrigerator and dishwasher once a month and as needed.
   b. Wash windows twice a year and as needed.
   c. Clean and dust closets and cupboards twice a year and as needed.
3. Laundry
4. Ironing
5. Light mending
6. Start supper
7. Grocery shopping
8. Miscellaneous light errands (i.e., dry cleaning)
9. Other duties as given by Drs. Jones or Smith

Work begins late July-early August (baby due 7/1)

Hours: 7:30 a.m. to 5:00 or 6:00 p.m., when one parent arrives home.
-- One Saturday morning a month 7:30 a.m.-2:00 p.m.
-- Not on most Thursdays
-- One half the office holidays (when Dr. Jones is on call)

Personal days off: two weeks a year with 2-week advance notice

Job Evaluation: Every six months with raise consideration every year.

I have received a copy of the job description and have reviewed and read with Dr. Jones the listed responsiblities.

_____   _____
Applicant Name   Date

References

Angel M. Juggling a personal and professional life. J Am Med Wom Assoc 1982; 37(3):64-68.

Avery M. Women in medicine, 1979: What are the issues? J Am Med Wom Assoc 1981;35:79-82.

Battle CU. Working and motherhood: A view of today's realities. J Am Med Wom Assoc 1985;40(3):74-76.

Baucum-Copeland, et al. Pregnant resident: Career conflict? J Am Med Wom Assoc 1983;38(4):103-105.

Bell DM, Gleiber DW, Mercer AA, et al. Illness associated with child daycare: A study of incidence and cost. Am J Public Health 1989;79(4):479-484.

Bernstein AE. Maternity leave for housestaff: Moving from advocacy to advice. J Am Med Wom Assoc 1988;43(3):85-88.

Deitch SR, Ed. Health in daycare: A manual for health professionals. American Academy of Pediatrics, Elk Grove Village, IL, 1987.

Endsley RC, Bradbard MR. Quality daycare. Prentice-Hall, Inc., Englewood Cliffs, NJ, 1981.

Heins M. Women physicians. Radcliff Quarterly June 1979, p. 11-14.

Heins M, Smack S, et al. A profile of the woman physician. J Am Med Wom Assoc 1977;32(11):421-427.

Heins M, Stillman B, et al. Attitudes of pediatricians towards maternal employement. Pediatrics 1983;72(3):283-290.

Hoffman L. Effect on children of working mothers. Hoffman L, Nye FI, ed. Jossey-Bass, San Francisco, 1974.

Howell M. The impact of working on mother and child: What are the facts? J Am Med Wom Assoc 1985;40(3):84-88.

Indiana Administrative Code. 470 IAC 3-3-71 Rule #4.

Kamerman S. The child care debate: Working mothers versus America. Working Woman November 1983, p. 131.

Kaplan H. Women physicians--The more effective recruitment and utilization of their talents and their resistance to it. The Woman Physician 1970;25(9):561-570.

Kebschull S. Group for N.C. working women to focus on childcare, pay equity. Winston-Salem Journal, June 17, 1989, page 8.

Konanc J. What support groups for women students do: A retrospective inquiry. J Am Med Wom Assoc 1979;34:275-282.

Medica Survey. Medica Fall 1983, p. 4-5.

Nadelson C, Notman M. Child psychiatry prospectives: Women, work, and children. J Am Acad Child Psychiatry 1981;20:863-875.

Nadelson C, Notman M, Lowenstein P. The practice patterns, lifestyles and stresses of women and men entering medicine: A follow-up study of Harvard Medical School graduates from 1967 to 1977. J Am Med Wom Assoc 1979;34(11): 400-406.

National Survey on Family Childcare, September, 1983; Gallup Poll.

Potter RL. Resident, woman, wife, mother: Issues for women in training. J Am Med Wom Assoc 1983;38(4):101-102.

Rapoport R, Rapoport R. Further considerations on a dual-career family. Human Relations 1971;24(6):519-533.

Rippis AK. Medicine & motherhood. Am Med News February 24, 1989, p. 35-38.

Scharff JS. Understanding and satisfying the psychological needs of infants and toddlers. J Am Med Wom Assoc 1985;40(3):77-79.

Scher M, Benedek E, et al. Psychiatrist-Wife-Mother: Some aspects of role integration. Am J Psychiatry 1976;133(7):830-834.

Scott N. The balancing act. Universal Press Syndicate, Kansas City, 1978.

Sinal S, Weavil P, Camp MG. Child care choices of women physicians. J Am Med Wom Assoc 1989;44(6):183-184.

Stein BA, Leventhal SE. Psychopathology in adolescent children of physicians. Can Med Assoc J 1984;130:599-602.

Steketee RW, Reid S, Cheng T, et al. Recurrent outbreaks of giardiasis in a child daycare center, Wisconsin. Am J Public Health 1989;79(4):485-490.

Stewart DE, Robinson GE. Combining motherhood with psychiatric training and practice. Can J Psychiatry 1985;30(1):28-34.

Wasserman RC, Hassuk BM, Young PC, Land ML. Health care of physicians' children. Pediatrics 1989;83(3):319-322.

Winter R. Course helps future M.D.'s balance career, family life. Am Med News March 11, 1983, p 26.

Women M.D.'s join the fight. Med World News October 23, 1970, p. 22-28.

Zylke JW. Day-care quality and quantity become challenges for parents, politicians, and medical researchers. JAMA 1988;260(22):3247-3249.

Zylke JW. Among latchkey children problems: Insufficient day-care facilities, data on possible harm. JAMA 1988;260(23):3399-3400.

13
Stress Prevention and Management

Stress is the way of life--a condition that is only compounded by an individual being a physician. One solution to the dilemma of managing stress lies in prevention. Some proponents of this method have suggested prescreening medical school applicants for ability to handle stress and teaching values clarification during medical school (Spears). Others have suggested making support groups, stress management techniques and methods for early identification of problems during medical training a part of every medical school (Hoferik, Gerber).

Dealing with the problems and stresses of being a physician is not easy. There continues to be a macho attitude underlying the commonly held view that internships and residencies should be trials by ordeal. Until this basic underlying attitude changes, it will be difficult to address the stresses of medical training. In the meantime, courses or workshops in primary prevention techniques such as stress recognition, stress management and interpersonal skills could be highly beneficial for medical students, residents, and, in the long run, physicians.

The literature is long on identifying the problems of physician stress and impairment, but short on adequate solutions (Spears). Although about one in five Fortune 500 companies has developed some sort of stress management program for their top-level executives (Walis), this would appear impractical for the individual physician or the under-funded medical school.

There is no single approach to stress management that is right for everyone--as the response to stress varies widely, so does the treatment. However, the same advice that physicians give patients for identifying stress and learning to respond adaptively is applicable to physicians themselves (Spears): one person may need a prescription for exercise and time off, while another may need psychotherapy.

The first step to stress management in any situation, however, is recognition of stress, coupled with knowledge of one's own positive and negative coping mechanisms. There are several specific basic stress reduction techniques, but physicians in particular need to address time management, relaxation techniques, social support, support groups, professional counseling, and the choice of the best practice alternative. Prevention of stress through incorporating stress management techniques into everyday life is of ultimate importance.

Recognition of Stress

It seems to be very difficult for professionals to recognize and especially to admit that stress may be affecting them and their health. But by watching for the effects of stress, it is possible to take early corrective action to prevent impairment. The signs of stress are classic, but vary from person to person. Thus, each individual needs to know her/his own stress 'cues'. The person affected may develop headaches, a stiff neck or nagging backache. The person may be irritable and intolerant of even minor disturbances by other people. The temper seems to flair and yelling at others without cause becomes a problem. The heart rate usually increases with stress and a feeling of exhaustion even after a good night's sleep is common. Recognizing these as signs of stress is the first step in combating it (Jasmine).

Using a stress scale is another method for recognition of stresses. A popular one is that of psychiatrists Thomas Holmes and Richard Rahle called the "Holmes-Rahle Scale of Social Readjustment" (see Table 13-1) which rates the impact of life events as stressors. The psychiatrists' research (Holmes) showed that in a sample of 88 young physicians, the young physician with a score of 300 or more on the scale, had a 70% chance of suffering from ulcers, psychiatric disturbances, broken bones or other health problems within the ensuing two years. Those who scored under 200 had only a 37% chance of such illness. The Holmes-Rahle Scale of Social Readjustment has proven to be an effective prognosticator of stress-related illnesses (Walis). Reviewing this scale and its indicators of stress can be useful for the physician.

Another method for stress recognition is identification of one's own personality characteristics that have been associated with a likelihood of increased stress. The scale, "Personality Risk Factors for Stress," provides an assessment of the aspects of one's personality that could lead to stress. Factors indicating a high likelihood should give one pause for thought as to their importance in one's life (Table 13-2).

Recognition of Positive and Negative Coping Mechanisms

The next step in stress management is consideration of one's personal coping mechanisms. Consider whether or not they are positive or negative: do they reduce the cause or response to the stress or do they only reduce the short-term stress at the expense of long-term problems? Are they

TABLE 13-1 Social Readjustment Rating Scale*

Event	Value
Death of Spouse	100
Divorce	73
Marital separation	65
Jail term	63
Death of close family member	63
Personal injury or illness	53
Marriage	50
Fired from work	47
Marital reconciliation	45
Retirement	45
Change in family member's health	44
Pregnancy	40
Sex difficulties	39
Addition to family	39
Business readjustment	39
Change in financial status	38
Death of close friend	37
Change to different line of work	36
Change in number of marital arguments	35
Mortgage or loan over $10,000	31
Foreclosure of mortgage or loan	30
Change in work responsibilities	29
Son or daughter leaving home	29
Trouble with in-laws	29
Outstanding personal achievement	28
Spouse begins or stops work	26
Starting or finishing school	26
Change in living conditions	25
Revision of personal habits	24
Trouble with boss	23
Change in work hours, conditions	20
Change in residence	20
Change in schools	20
Change in recreational habits	19
Change in church activities	19
Change in social activities	18
Mortgage or loan under $10,000	17
Change in sleeping habits	16
Change in number of family gatherings	15
Change in eating habits	15
Vacation	13
Christmas season	12
Minor violation of the law	11

Scoring		
300+	90%	chance of serious illness within the next year
150-300	51%	chance of getting ill in the next two years.
0-150	37%	chance of getting ill in the next two years.

*Reprinted with permission from Med World News June 11, T. Holmes and R. Rahle, Women Physicians, 1979, Pergamon Press, Ltd.

TABLE 13-2 Personal Risk Analysis for Stress for Women Physicians

		Yes	No
1.	Is maintaining your superwoman image all important?		
2.	Do you let your practice take control of your life?		
3.	Are your family's and patient's needs more important than your own?		
4.	Do you feel overloaded all the time?		
5.	Do you blame others for your problems?		
6.	Is it hard for you to delegate work at home and at the office?		
7.	Do you find it difficult to change behaviors?		
8.	Are you waiting for someone else to help reduce your stress?		
9.	Do you receive positive feedback outside of work on your 'mother' role?		
10.	Do you continually strive to achieve?		
11.	Are you considered too intense?		
12.	Do you have lack support from friends and family?		

Count the Number of Yes Responses:

0 - 3	Minimal risk
4 - 8	Moderate risk
9 - 12	Significant risk

adaptive or maladaptive? Positive mechanisms are described in further detail below. Negative coping mechanisms are discussed in the chapter on Physician Stress.

There appear to be a number of personality characteristics that are effective in coping. Among them are (Walis, McLean):

1. A sense of being in control of one's life;
2. The ability to change and be flexible;
3. Optimism--the attitude that there is hope in most circumstances; and
4. A deep commitment to some goal or belief.

A similar concept called 'hardiness' is described by Barnett (1987), with hardiness combining commitment (to something one is doing), control (actions and belief that one can influence outcome), and challenge (belief that change is normative) (p. 322).

The type of coping style is also important. Blake and Vandiver (1988) found that an active-cognitive style of coping was positively and avoidance-coping was negatively associated with health status.

Active-cognitive coping included such things as: trying to see the positive side; trying to step back from the situation and to be more objective; praying for guidance or strength; taking things one step at a time; considering several alternatives for handling the problem, and drawing on past experiences (recognition of dealing with a similar situation before).

Attempting to block stress-producing beliefs through positive self-statements (such as those based on the above active-cognitive coping style) and positive imagery is called stress inoculation (King).

Overall, Barnett (1987) concludes that "the more women feel in control, have high self-esteem and low self-denigration, are Type B rather than Type A, and express hardiness, the less likely are they to fall ill under stress." (p. 325)

Basic Stress Reducing Techniques

There has been a lot written about management of stress, but most of the basic techniques appear to be simply good, plain sense (Walis, Jasmine, Murphy, King):

1. Keep your weight to its ideal level.
2. Don't smoke.
3. Don't use caffeine.
4. Exercise regularly.
5. Take time out for yourself regularly and relax.
6. Participate in activities outside of work, particularly hobbies.
7. Avoid stressful situations. Although this is practically impossible, do avoid unnecessary stressful situations.
8. Plan in advance to make a known situation less stressful.
9. Decide if an issue is worth the stress. Changed expectations greatly reduces stress.

Career Patterns

One common solution to role strain for women physicians has been to back off from ambition. Another is to play wonderwoman and hang on to all of the old domestic roles while pursuing a career full-blast. The negative affects of this are obvious--extreme role strain, fatigue, anxiety and resentment of having too much work to do and never enough time (Dowling). There are three basic options in terms of career patterns for women faced with the roles of mother, wife, and physician as described by Rapoport (1971):

1. *Conventional*--In this pattern, the woman drops her career when she marries or after childbearing and concentrates on being a housewife and mother with no intention of returning to work. This is unusual for women physicians.
2. *Interrupted*--In this pattern, the woman drops out of work for a period of time when her children are small with all intentions of returning to work. Several pilot projects for retraining of inactive physicians have been successful in permitting women to re-enter active medical practice (Brown, Wineberg), but they remain few and far between.
3. *Continuous*--In this pattern, the woman interrupts her work only minimally or not at all for childbearing. This is the model into which the 'superwoman,' as well as others, fit.

Each of these is a viable option with its own pros and cons depending upon an individual woman's situation.

Recently, Cartwright (1987) has described what she calls "role montage," essentially the complexities of changing patterns and priorities over the lifetime of a woman's career development and the changing nature of the demands of the roles over time.

There has been little support for the multiple roles of women in medicine. If the woman physician does decide to combine motherhood and marriage with medicine, she needs to adopt the philosophy that these roles are indeed compatible, and simultaneously her right. Symonds (1979) claims that women do not believe they are entitled to achieve--a significant inhibitor to the achievement in itself. She has found that women have serious difficulties nurturing their own inner growth and development. Younger women appear to be growing up with a healthier sense of entitlement to all that life can offer and hopefully this will continue to grow as more women enter medicine.

Techniques for Reducing Role Strain

There are several techniques for reducing role strain:

1. *"Role cycling"*--allowing yourself to give higher priority to one or another role at different times.
2. *Subjective rationalization*--attributing one's actions to rational and creditable motives regardless of the unconscious reasons; for example, believing that it is not the quantity of time you spend with your children, but the quality of time that is important to their well-being.

3. *Changed expectations*--learning to develop a flexible attitude toward daily problems. For example, teaching children to be more self-reliant and independent or letting the housework go. Learn to develop a flexible attitude toward daily problems.
4. *Decreased confrontation with societal norms*--avoiding situations which highlight differences with others. For example, dual-career couples can choose friends with similar backgrounds, thus reducing conflict (Rapoport).
5. *Creative child care.* As noted in the Child Care Chapter, stress and role strain are less when the parent is comfortable with the childcare arrangements.
6. *Hire help!!* Decrease role strain by hiring help, probably several kinds: hire someone to take care of the children, to mow and landscape the yard, fix the car, do the housework, bring the groceries to your house. You can even hire someone to select and purchase clothes for you. While hiring costs money, health and happiness are more important. It has been said that what all women physicians need is a good wife!

Time Management (Table 13-3)

Stress is not avoidable. Like it or not, each individual will need to identify the personal stresses affecting her/his life. The following time analysis is the starting point for listing personal stress factors. The first step in organizing a time management system is setting priorities. Ask yourself, what is most important to you? What is it that you want to? After considering this and filling in the form, list how you feel about the findings. This analysis provides the master plan for instituting a new time priority program. Recognition is the beginning of the resolution. The rest of the solution is dedication to the commitment. If physical exercise is important, for instance, a schedule must be adhered to that allocates time for the activity. If a busy physician waits until she has time, the time will never come.

Relaxation Techniques

Relaxation is a natural method for coping with stress. Relaxation should allow you to rest your body and mind from stress. Most people consider relaxing to be an evening of television, but sometimes the stress of a football game, for example, puts emotions on a slow boil. That which is relaxing for one person may not be relaxing for another. Relaxation can be found in a great variety of activities. To be relaxing, it must allow the

TABLE 13-3 Time Analysis

Calculate the approximate amount of time spent per week on the categories listed. Recalculate the desired hours on the right-handlist.

Time Spent in These Activities	Actual Hours/Week	Desired Hours/Week
Work		
Sleeping		
Eating		
Commuting		
Parent/child interaction		
Spouse interaction		
Food preparation		
Shopping		
Housework		
Recreation		
Physical exercise		
Other		

mind to slow down and release those things that cause stress. True relaxing is an acquired skill. Learned relaxation techniques, including meditation, biofeedback, progressive relaxation and exercise, are valuable, positive coping mechanisms.

Meditation Meditation is a term applied to the state of prolonged focusing on a word, subject or object. If the focus is on an object, the eyes remain open, but otherwise are closed. Meditation is usually done in the sitting position with a quiet atmosphere and may use as a focus specific bodily functions such as heart rate or breathing (McLean).

The first popular therapeutic relaxation was transcendental meditation (TM) (Walis). Physiological studies have shown that TM can produce marked changes in the body, called the relaxation response, including a decrease in heart rate, a lowering of blood pressure and a reduction in oxygen consumption. If done 10-20 minutes once or twice a day, it has been shown to produce a lasting reduction in stress-related symptoms.

Biofeedback Biofeedback is a simple process of monitoring one or more of the bodily functions with electrical devices that translate the activity into a receivable signal. The theory of biofeedback rests on the assumption that once a person can observe this message, she/he can learn to control the function being monitored. The use of biofeedback is a rapidly expanding field and many mail-order catalogues today contain instruments for home use. The devices are able to measure a variety of responses, including blood pressure, body temperature, muscle tension, and the galvanic skin response (McLean).

Progressive Relaxation A process similar to biofeedback is called progressive relaxation. This process is based on the assumption that stress and anxiety are directly related to muscle tension. If stress caused the tightness of muscles the relaxation of these muscles should reduce stress (McLean). Progressive relaxation is usually attempted in a reclining position in a quiet room. It can take many hours of learning the exercises to become adept at rapid and complete progressive relaxation.

Exercise Exercise has been mentioned frequently as a stress reducer. Its importance in an overall stress reduction program cannot be over-emphasized. Exercise is a means of relaxation, but must obviously be tailored to the individual and her/his health. Exercise can be viewed as a natural response to the fight or flight reaction. Stress primes the body for action, and exercise expends the build-up energy. An added benefit of exercising regularly is cardiovascular fitness, which contributes to overall well-being. Studies have shown regular exercise to be an adjunctive therapy in the treatment of depression and hypertension (McLean).

Support Groups

Support groups have been mentioned several times in recommendations for stress reduction and a fair amount has been written about their benefits, particularly to women medical students (Wineberg, Davidson, Konanc). Groups have been found to be of great benefit in increasing the capacity of women students and residents to deal with hostility and to help establish sustained friendships (Davidson). Formalized groups in medical school have brought enduring relationships among women classmates and increased their understanding of women's professional difficulties (Konanc). As a result of group experience, there is usually an increased feeling of closeness and solidarity in the working arena. This has been accompanied by decreased feelings of threat and competitiveness. Outside of the group experience, there is usually a decrease in the use of negative coping mechanisms and an increase in the use of positive coping mechanisms (Kahn).

Social Support

As noted by Blake and Vandiver (1988), social supports have a positive, direct effect on health. "Four prospective population-based studies have found higher mortality during follow-up periods ranging from 30 months to 12 years in adults with weak as compared to strong supports. . . . Several studies have found increased rates of psychological impairment, particularly depression, in people with poor supports." (Blake)   Both intimate, confiding relationships and acquaintances are important, with the intimate ones more important to health status (Belle). While this does not prove that increasing social supports in times of stress will improve the individual's outcome, it would appear that increased contacts with other individuals, family and others can have an ameliorating affect on perceived stress and a positive impact on health.

Women clearly participate in more and larger social support networks (Cleary). They tend to have more confidants, whereas men have fewer confidants and more casual acquaintances (Belle).   Though these attachments are generally positive, women's larger networks may produce additional strains when individuals in the network turn to them for support and help (Belle) as women are much more likely to accept a call to help others (Wethington). For example, an ill relative requiring substantial help with daily activities can be a source of stress.   The stress of the social networks, however, is greater for women with fewer other resources, such as education and money (Belle). In other words, a larger support network was only helpful to women with a fair amount of other resources, which would generally be true of women physicians.

Thus, women's tendency toward intimate friendships and social contact may have a protective effect on health.

Religion

Craigie et al (1988), through reviewing the literature, believe that active involvement in a religion is associated with decreased morbidity and better physical and mental health. This effect may occur because of a variety of things, such as religious proscription of detrimental behaviors, increased levels of social support and/or commitment to a major life goal. Regardless of the mechanism, religion can be an important tool for stress prevention and management for many people.

Professional Counseling

Even with the help of the above-mentioned intervention techniques, some people will find themselves without the personal resources to cope successfully with the stress of their profession and personal life. If the physician is unable to learn sufficient coping techniques, she/he should consider psychoanalysis or supportive psychotherapy. Physicians often fear obtaining professional help, but they should not hesitate to do so in order to prevent impairment.

Shared-Schedule Residencies

In 1976, Section 709 of the Health Professions Education Assistance Act mandated shared-schedule positions in residency programs for family practice, general internal medicine, and general pediatrics in institutions receiving Federal assistance (Shapiro 1979). This was rescinded under the Reagan budget cuts in the summer of 1983 (Shapiro 1980). There are, however, a variety of shared-schedule options that currently are available.

According to Section 709, a shared position was defined as a program which is shared by two individuals in which each individual:

1. Engaged in at least two-thirds, but no more than three-fourths of the total training prescribed for such a position;
2. Received the amount of credit for certification in the medical specialty for which the position provides training, which is equal to the amount of training, engaged in such a year;
3. Received at least half the salary; and
4. Received all of the benefits.

There are four general types of shared-schedule residencies (Shapiro 1978). These include:

1. *The Integrated Continuing Model* In this model, two residents are paired in one training slot. This is a prototype and follows the original guidelines set by the government. Both residents will work between two-thirds and three-quarters time and night and weekend call would be divided on an alternating schedule.
2. *Alternating Time Blocks* One resident may be on for six month and off for six months. There may be various lengths of time involved.
3. *Night Float* In this system, one of the residents is on night duty while the other resident is on during the day.
4. *Variable Schedule* This is any combination of the above models.

In one study (Shapiro 1980), 1,735 institutions were surveyed, with 85% responding. Less than one-third (28.9%) reported options for some type of reduced schedule training in at least one specialty. The total number of programs with such options was 1,051. The reduced schedule training by special arrangement was by far the most popular among the program directors. The least popular was the night float option. In primary care fields, the integrated continuing model is the only viable alternative assuring continuity of patient care as well as full participation by the residents in the formal educational activities of the programs.

According to Brunton and Ostergaard (1982), 15% of directors of family practice residency programs would be willing to consider offering flexible time programs. The directors perceived the desire for flexible scheduling as a women's problem. The directors predicted 14% of the male or female housestaff would want more time for their families. In actuality, 59% of male and 84% of female medical students thought they would want a flexible time program (Brunton). Crowley (quoted in Greganti) said that 11% of all, and 24% of internal medicine residencies, offer shared-schedule programs. Obviously there is an enormous gap between medical student interests and the availability of flexible residencies.

It must be noted that there are problems with shared-schedule residencies:

1. Concern about continuity of patient services (Brunton, Shapiro 1978).
2. Concern about the quality of education received by the residents in such a situation. In order to provide first class training, the housestaff must be able to participate in all educational situations offered (Shapiro 1978).
3. The shared-schedule residency is a financial burden on a medical institution because of having to provide full benefits for residents theoretically working only half-time (Shapiro 1978).
4. There is resentment, envy and often open hostility by the full-time housestaff toward residents who are doing shared-time programs (Heins, Shapiro 1978).
5. Many participating residents often are actually working 3/4 time but receiving 1/2 pay.
6. The schedule obviously leads to significant delay in completion of training.

On the other hand, there may be some benefits to the directors of medical programs who offer shared-schedule residencies. For example, 1. a more interesting type of person might be attracted to medicine. In one survey (Brunton), the directors stated that they might indeed find more experienced, more intelligent and responsible housestaffs through shared-schedule flexible programs. 2. Housestaff morale, in general, might improve. 3. The ultimate benefactor might be society when the young physicians are given the opportunity to satisfactorily develop their personal and professional life (Brunton).

Practice Alternatives

The practice environment is a very important part of the solution to role strain and stress for the woman physician. There is very little written in the literature on the various practice styles available, but several less well known, but feasible, styles known to be in use will be discussed here. The commonly discussed practice types, which attract many men and women, would include solo practice, group or partnership practice, institutional practice, and academia. Less frequently discussed styles, which may be particularly pertinent to women, include shared or part-time positions, the home office, the 'child in the office,' practice with spouse, and combinations of the above. Each will be briefly described here:

Shared or Part-time Positions With a shared position, each physician shares an equivalent percentage of the patient load and time in the office. An example would be two physicians scheduling themselves to see patients, one in the morning, one in the afternoon. That way each works 1/2 time with a practice equivalent to one solo practitioner. Physicians can also work parttime, with the same schedule each week or alternating time arrangements, such as alternating six months working and six months not working. The major disadvantage to part-time positions is that the overhead and benefits are often a greater proportion of the income. To receive full-time benefits while working part-time requires proportionately more money. Few malpractice insurance companies permit part-time physicians to pay reduced rate premiums.

Home Office The home office arrangement tends to be opted for only by the solo practitioner. A woman usually chooses this option for the convenience of being near home. However, the privacy of the physician is distinctly decreased because of the presence of patients and personnel in the home. There is also isolation from the rest of the medical community because of the location of the practice. However, it is a reasonable and viable alternative for many women, particularly psychiatrists. It is also more common than many realize--a recent report noted there were more than 100 home offices in Montgomery County, Maryland, alone (Voelker)!

Child in the Office Women physicians who have the opportunity to do so may opt to take their small children with them to the office. The usual arrangement is to have one exam room or office be the child's playroom. Job descriptions for office personnel would include child care responsibilities. This allows for mother-child interaction whenever there is a free moment and is convenient for breast feeding. This works best in a solo office situation and when the child is very young.

Practice with Spouse This option is not commonly chosen, but allows for whatever time constraints the couple decides is necessary for each individual. The biggest problem with this arrangement is coverage for call. Unless other physicians are actively taking call, there is no time for the couple to be away together.

In the authors' experience, women frequently find practicing with other women more congenial than practicing with men. Women more frequently have similar practice styles and beliefs, such as how much time to spend with patients and how to charge. Other women may be more tolerant of the requirements of motherhood. More women than men are interested in these alternative practice arrangements.

Summary

The preceding chapters have provided a discussion on the nature of stress and its affect on a person's life. Hopefully, each individual will be able to identify her/his own personal stresses and the importance of these stresses to their lives. After a personal evaluation, each person must desire to change their stress level and their response in order to develop a realistic plan to follow. Specific stress reducing activities and options--a number of which are briefly outlined here--must be incorporated into daily life in order to successfully manage stress.

References

Barnett RC, Biener L, Baruch GK, eds.   Gender & Stress.   The Free Press, Macmillan, Inc., New York, 1987.

Belle D. Gender differences in the social moderators of stress. In Gender & Stress, Barnett RC, Biener L, Baruch GK, eds., The Free Press, Macmillan, Inc., New York, 1987, p. 257-277.

Blake RL, Vandiver TA. The association of health with stressful life changes, social supports, and coping. Fam Pract Res J 1988;7(4):205-218.

Brown M, Sakai J, et al. A retraining program for inactive physicians. West J Med November 1969:396-399.

Brunton SM, Ostergaard D. Report on a workshop on maternity and paternity leave held at the Directors of Family Practice Residency Programs Workshop, 1982.

Cartwright LK. Role montage: Life patterns of professional women. J Am Med Wom Assoc 1987;42(5):142-148.

Cleary PD. Gender differences in stress-related disorders. In Gender & Stress, Barnett RC, Biener L, Baruch GK, eds. The Free Press, Macmillan, Inc., New York, 1987, p. 39 - 72.

Craigie FC, Liu IY, Larson DB, Lyons JS. A systematic analysis of religious variables in the Journal of Family Practice 1976-1986. J Fam Pract 1988;27(5):509-513.

Davidson V. Coping styles of women medical students. J Med Educ 1978;53: 902-907.

Dowling C. Cinderella complex. Simon & Schuster, New York,1981.

Gerber L. Married to their careers. Tavistock Publications, New York, 1983.

Greganti MA, Fletcher SW. House staff pregnancy in internal medicine residencies. Ann Intern Med 1985;102(1):123-125.

Heins M, Smack S, Martindale L, et al. Comparison of productivity of women and men physicians. JAMA 1977;237(23):2514-2517.

Hoferik M, Sarnowski S. Feelings of loneliness in medical students. J Med Educ 1981;56:397-403.

Holmes PH, Rahle RH. Social Readjustment Rating Scale. J Psychosomatic Research. Elmsford, New York, Pergamon Press, 1967;11:216.

Kahn N, Schaeffer H. A process group approach to stress reduction and personal growth in a family practice residency program. J Fam Pract 1981;12(6):1043-1047.

King M, Stanley G, Burrows G. Stress: Theory and practice. Grune & Stratton, Orlando, FL, 1987.

Konanc J. What support groups for women medical students do: A retrospective inquiry. J Am Med Wom Assoc 1979;34:282.

Jasmine S, Hill L, et al. The art of managing stress. Nursing June 1981, 53-57.

McLean A. Work Stress. Addison-Wesley Publishing Co, Reading, MA, 1982, p. 27-99.

Murphy M. Stress management classes as a health promotion tool. A Canadian Nurse June 1981, p. 29-31.

Rapoport R, Rapoport R. Further considerations of a dual-career family. Human Relations 1971;24(6):519-533.

Shapiro E, Driscoli S. Part-time residencies versus shared scheduling. Resident and Staff Physician, December 1978, p. 66-71.

Shapiro E, Driscoli S. Shared schedule training: Compliance with section 709, P.L. 94-484. J Med Educ 1979;54:576-578.

Shapiro E, Lane M, et al. The supply of reduced schedule residencies. J Am Med Wom Assoc 1980;35(2):42-50.

Spears B. A time management system for preventing physician impairment. J Fam Pract 1981;13:175-180.

Symonds A. The wife as the professional. Am J Psychoanalysis 1979;39(1):552-563.

Voelker R. MDs fear laws may limit home offices. Am Med News May 26, 1989, p. 15-17.

Walis C. Stress--Can we cope? Time, June 6, 1983.

Wethington E, McLeod JD, Kessler RC. The importance of life events for explaining sex differences in psychological distress. In Gender & Stress, Barnett RC, Biener L, Baruch GK, eds. The Free Press, Macmillan, Inc., New York, 1987, p. 144-156.

Wineberg E. Retraining physicians. J Med Educ 1972;47:625-630.

14
The Future

Women physicians are becoming an increasingly larger proportion of the profession. In spite of greater numbers of women in medical schools, women will not reach 25% of the practicing physicians until the year 2020 (Pitts). Attitudes appear to be changing and there is considerable improvement in the place and role of women in medicine today. Even with such changes, it is important to remember the setbacks of the past. Major changes in attitudes and expectations must continue or women will be in danger of repeating the past cycle of events and, once again, decrease their numbers in medicine. Certainly, the increased numbers of women in medicine should benefit other women who are coming into the profession. There are few role models in the older generation, and women physicians today are still juggling their concurrent roles of mother, wife and physician. As the number of women physicians increases, modeling of these roles will be greater. Future women physicians will have less difficulty because of the adequacy and abundance of role models and advocates. Women should also feel less isolated and more at ease with a profession that has reasonable numbers of other women.

What about the possible impact of an expanding supply of women physicians? It would be very gratifying for women physicians to think they will make medicine more caring and humanistic, as is often conjectured. Women physicians do tend to be more oriented toward nurturing and to patient relationships than do men physicians. However, it is unlikely that women can alter this perceived lack of humanism in medicine by themselves. Such a major change will probably occur only if there is modified medical school admission criteria to reflect a desire for this characterisitic as well as change in the current reward system in medicine (Eisenberg). Though there is a possibility for a change in the amount of humanism in medicine in the future, it currently appears that changes will occur for reasons other than the gender of the physician (Heins), such as patient demands.

It is not clear what other differences might emerge with greater numbers of women physicians, although there are a variety of speculations. Concurrent with the increasing number of women in medicine, the United

States has been in the phase of rapid expansion in the numbers of physicians, possibly even creating an oversupply (GMENAC, Bowman). Some medical schools are cutting back on the number of admissions. Physicians are facing increasing competition, not only from other physicians, but from other kinds of alternative health care workers. The ratio of physicians to nonphysician health care workers is decreasing. Pressure to reduce high health care costs concurrent with the expanding supply of physicians has created expansion in multi-institutional structures, and an increased 'business-sense' in the world of medicine.

How will women fit into this changing medical milieu? Perhaps their preference for shorter residencies and shorter working hours will decrease the popularity of costly subspecialties (Relman), reduce the current perceived specialty imbalance and lower the cost of care. Women physicians have traditionally been more likely to take salaried jobs, and they may be more willing to participate in experimentation with different economic arrangements for medical practice. It has been suggested that the preference for salaried positions may promote the success of Health Maintenance Organizations and possibly dilute some of medicine's opposition to economic reform (Woman Physicians). Also, if women physicians continue to avoid medical organizations as they have in the past, organized medicine will find itself, in the near future, in a very difficult position, with less power in numbers (Relman).

Thus, some of the impact on society and on the medical field of additional women will be good. But what about the impact on women? If medical school admissions decrease, will the gains made by women again be cut short? Will the large number of women in medicine further erode the prestige of the profession (Gray), and create a backlash of anger and decreased opportunity for women by the male physicians in power? Will the competition in medicine affect women more negatively than men? If someone is out of a job, will it be the woman rather than the man? Remember that the numbers of women in medicine increased dramatically at the turn of the last century, concurrent with what was perceived as a physician oversupply. The gains made by women at that time were quickly erased. The one major advantage that women have now, that they did not have then, is Federal law, which prohibits discrimination on the basis of sex. Recent Supreme Court decisions, however, have eroded the potential impact of such laws. Although one can argue about how effective these laws have been in creating equality among the sexes, it is clear that having the law on one's side should make retaining the gains much easier than in the past when no such laws existed.

Solutions to all of the problems that affect women physicians are not immediately available and grasped, partially because of the great transitions that are occurring. Discriminatory behavior and thinking continue and are not easily erased. Women physicians will always have to prioritize and juggle various roles, but there will be more role models to help smooth the way. Women will be more accepted as physicians. In terms of the changes that are affecting the larger world of medicine, women physicians will share the pressures with men, though a differential impact on women physicians may occur. Meanwhile, the large group of women physicians that currently are forging ahead will have to develop new models using their intuition and imagination. The upcoming group of women physicians will probably come to be known as the "innovative transitional generation."

References

Bowman MA, Katzoff JM, Garrison LP, Wills J. Estimates of physician requirements for 1990 for the specialties of neurology, anesthesiology, nuclear medicine, pathology, physical medicine and rehabilitation, and radiology--A further application of the GMENAC methodology. JAMA 1983;250(19):2623-2627.

Eisenberg C. Women as physicians. J Med Educ 1983;58:534-541.

GMENAC. Summary report of the Graduate Medical Education National Advisory Committee, Volume I. Office of Graduate Medical Education, Health Resources Administration, U.S. Department of Health and Human Services Publication (HRA) 81-651, September 1980.

Gray C. How will the new wave of women graduates change the medical profession? Can Med Assoc J 1980123:798-804.

Heins M. Women physicians. Radcliff Quarterly June 1979, 11-14.

Pitts FN. Women medical students. Letter to the Editor. JAMA 1978;240(12): 1238-1239.

Relman AS. Here come the women. N Engl J Med 1980;302(22):1252-1253.

Women Physicians. Med World News June 11, 1979.

Index